DIABETES DIET COOKBOOK AFTER 50: *Delicious and easy recipes to help manage your blood sugar*

CAROL L. WILLIAMS

Table of content

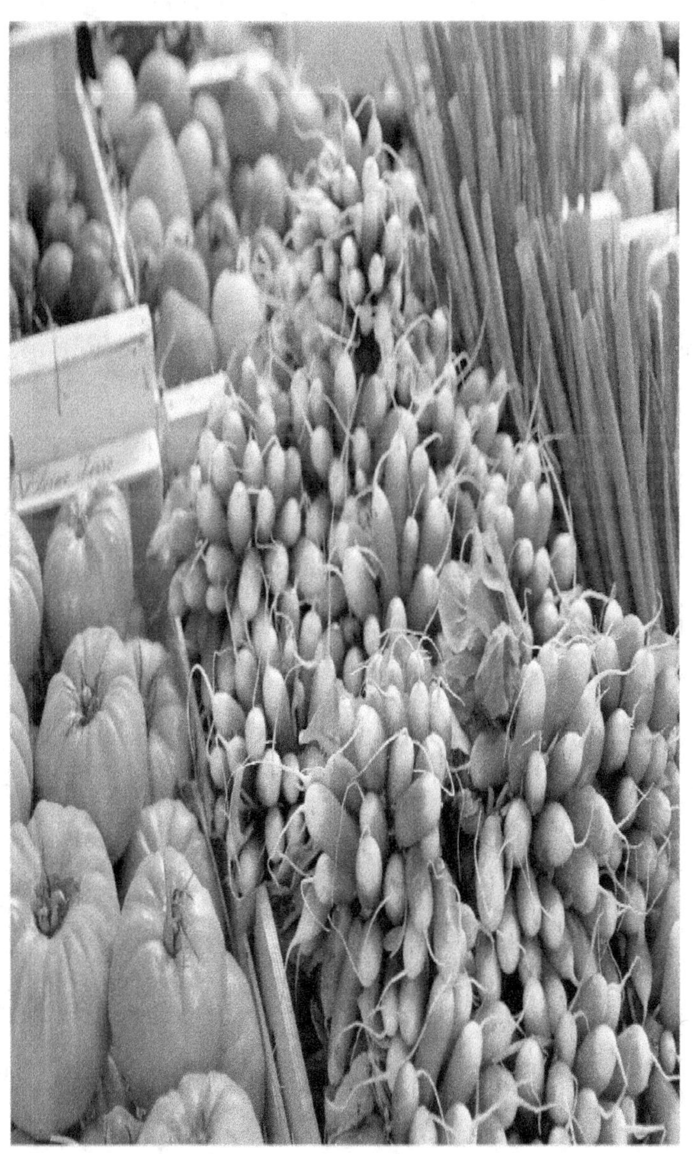

CHAPTER 1:

INTRODUCTION

Meet Karen, a 57-year-old lady with type 2 diabetes who was diagnosed five years ago. She had always been a foodie and relished in her favorite cuisine. But, after receiving the diagnosis, she realized she needed to make considerable adjustments to her food and lifestyle in order to keep her diabetes under control.

Karen initially struggled to accept her diagnosis, and it took some time for her to accept her condition. It was difficult for her to navigate the world of diabetes diets and meal preparation. Karen, on the other hand, started to make considerable dietary modifications with the assistance of her doctor and a trained dietician.

Karen's doctor stressed the need of a well-balanced diet in treating her diabetes. She needed to maintain a healthy weight, regulate her blood sugar levels, and lower her risk of diabetic complications. Karen was also recommended to cut down on carbohydrate consumption, increase fiber consumption, and consume a variety of nutrient-dense meals.

Karen worked with the dietician to develop a meal plan that included her favorite foods while still satisfying her nutritional needs. Karen discovered the importance of eating whole grains, lean proteins, healthy fats, and plenty of veggies and fruits. She also had to watch her portion sizes since eating too much may cause her blood sugar levels to skyrocket.

Karen's new meal plan took some getting accustomed to, but she eventually learned to make better eating choices. She began making her meals at home, using fresh and nutritious products. She also learnt to carefully read food labels and avoid meals with hidden sugars or bad fats.

Finding adequate substitutes for Karen's favorite recipes was one of the obstacles she encountered. She enjoyed spaghetti and bread, but she had to limit her carbohydrate consumption. She learned that through experimenting, she could still enjoy her favorite foods in moderation.

She discovered that whole-grain pasta and bread were good alternatives for white flour products. She also learnt how to regulate her portion sizes and to balance her carbohydrate consumption with protein and healthy fats.

Karen's new diet helped her regulate her blood sugar levels while also allowing her to lose weight gradually. She also began to feel more energy and had less desires for bad meals.

Karen began to exercise daily in addition to her new diet. She started walking, swimming, and doing yoga, which boosted her blood sugar levels and general wellness. She also learnt stress-reduction methods such as deep breathing, meditation, and mindfulness, which assisted her in being calm and focused.

Despite some setbacks, Karen was determined to get control of her diabetes and live a better lifestyle. She discovered that having a support system, which included her doctor, dietician, and family members, was critical in her journey.

She also joined a diabetic support group, which allowed her to connect with others who were going through similar circumstances.

Karen is pleased to report that she has been able to maintain a healthy weight, regulate her blood sugar levels, and lower her risk of diabetic complications. She maintains a healthy diet, exercises frequently, and takes her medicine as directed. She's also made certain lifestyle adjustments, such as cutting down on drinking and quitting smoking.

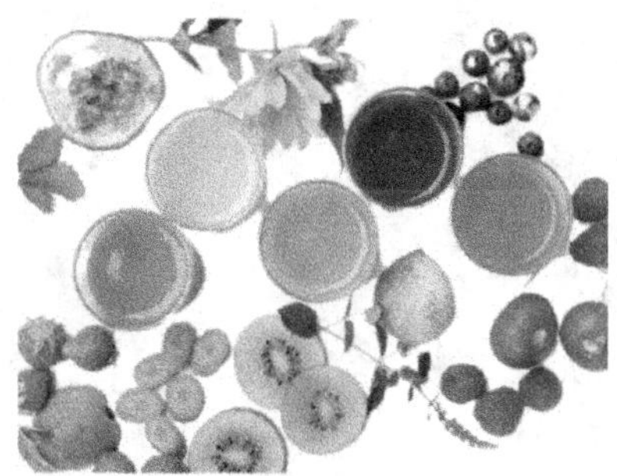

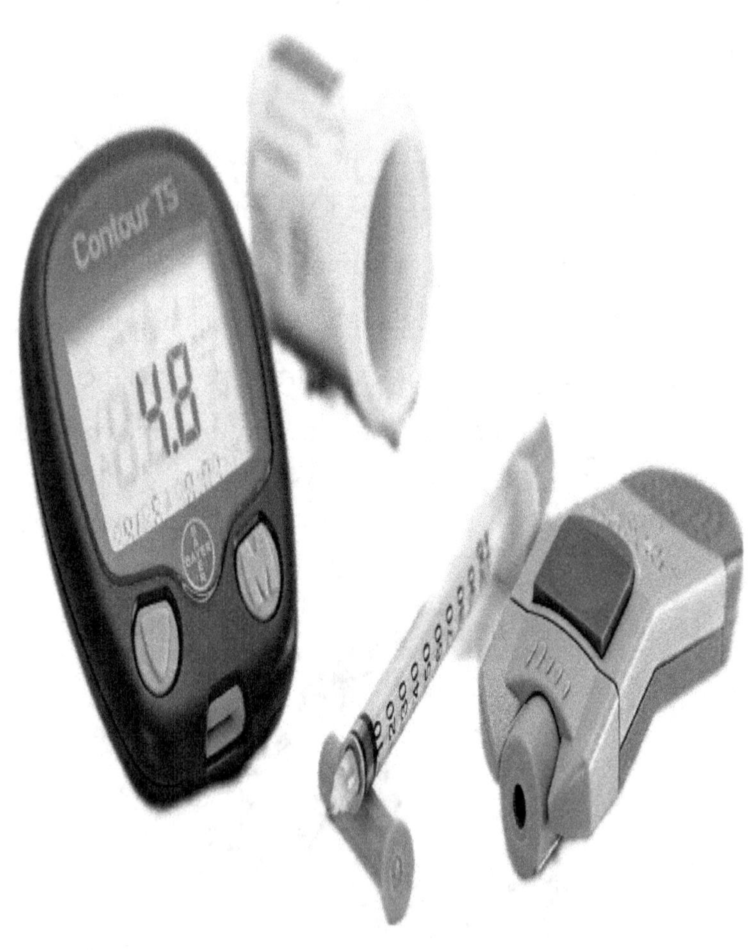

Contour TS
4.8

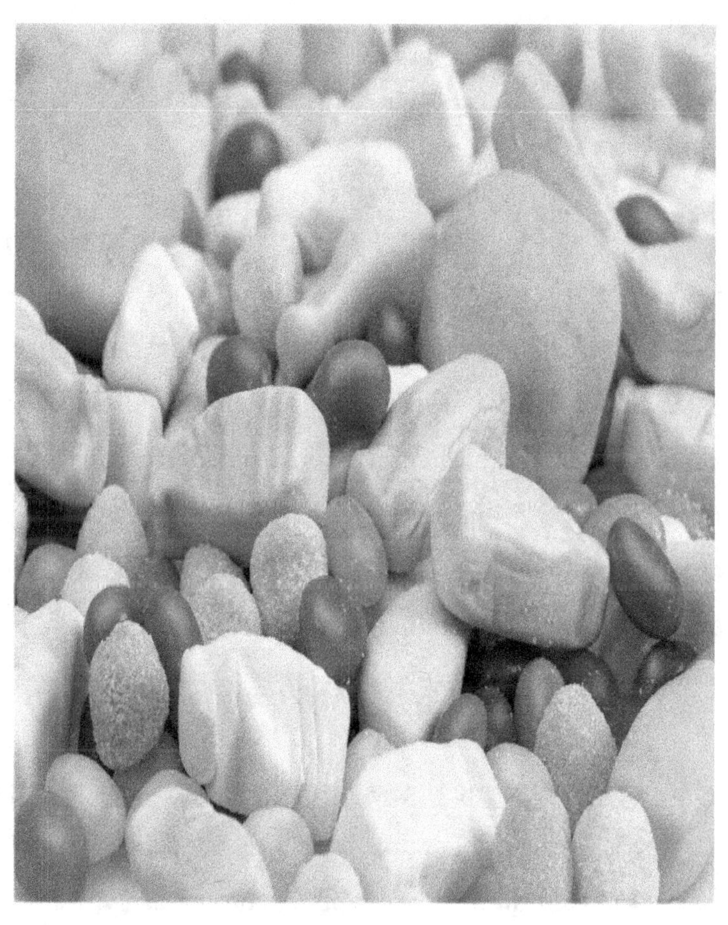

CHAPTER 2:

DIABETES AND AGING AN OVERVIEW

The Relationship Between Aging and Diabetes

The association between aging and diabetes beyond 50 is complicated and diverse, with a variety of physiological and behavioral variables contributing to the start and progression of the illness. As people age, they become more vulnerable to a variety of chronic illnesses, including diabetes, owing to a combination of hereditary and environmental factors.

Diabetes is a metabolic illness that affects the way the body uses glucose, the major source of energy for cells. The two primary kinds of diabetes are type 1 and type 2. Type 1 diabetes is an autoimmune illness that results in the loss of insulin-producing beta cells in the pancreas, whereas type 2 diabetes is a chronic condition that is caused by a combination of insulin resistance and beta cell failure.

As people age, their risk of getting type 2 diabetes rises owing to a number of variables, including changes in body composition, reduced physical activity, and modifications in hormone levels. According to the Centers for Disease Control and Prevention (CDC), over 25% of persons aged 65 and older have diabetes, with the great majority of cases having type 2 diabetes.

One of the key reasons leading to the increasing risk of type 2 diabetes with age is changes in body composition. As people age, they tend to undergo a progressive loss of muscular mass, known as sarcopenia, and an increase in body fat, especially in the stomach region. This alteration in body composition may lead to insulin resistance, a disease in which the body's cells become less receptive to insulin, the hormone that helps control blood glucose levels.

Insulin resistance is a major element in the development of type 2 diabetes, since it limits the body's capacity to properly utilise glucose for energy. Over time, this may lead to high blood glucose levels, which can cause a variety of issues, including cardiovascular illness, nerve damage, and kidney damage.

Another factor contributing to the increasing risk of type 2 diabetes with age is reduced physical activity. As people age, they tend to become less active, which might lead to weight gain and insulin resistance. Regular exercise is an essential approach to maintain muscle mass, enhance insulin sensitivity, and minimize the incidence of type 2 diabetes.

Hormone changes also play a role in the aging-diabetes association. Individuals' levels of insulin-like growth factor 1 (IGF-1) and sex hormones such as estrogen and testosterone fall as they age. These hormonal changes have the potential to influence glucose metabolism and lead to insulin resistance.

Apart from these physiological aspects, lifestyle factors such as nutrition and stress may also influence the association between aging and diabetes. Chronic stress may promote inflammation and affect glucose metabolism, while a diet heavy in refined carbs and saturated fats can contribute to insulin resistance and raise the risk of type 2 diabetes.

Diabetes prevention and management in older individuals need a multifaceted strategy that tackles these and other variables. Lifestyle therapies such as regular exercise, a balanced diet, and stress management strategies may be included, as well as medical interventions such as drugs to enhance glucose control and blood pressure management.

The Significance Of a Balanced Diet For Diabetic Elderly Persons

A balanced diet is essential for treating diabetes in those over the age of 50. A healthy diet helps to manage blood sugar levels, lower the risk of diabetic complications, and preserve general health and well-being. In this post, we will address the importance of a balanced diet for diabetes older people over the age of 50, including what to eat, what to avoid, and meal management suggestions.

What exactly is a balanced diet?

A well-balanced diet contains foods from all of the main dietary categories. This includes the following:

Fruits and vegetables are rich in vitamins, minerals, and fiber and should make up a substantial portion of any well-balanced diet.

 Consuming a variety of fruits and vegetables may help to lower the risk of chronic illnesses including diabetes, heart disease, and cancer.

Whole grains: Whole grains are high in fiber, which helps to manage blood sugar levels and support digestive health. Whole wheat, oats, quinoa, and brown rice are examples of whole grains.

Lean proteins, such as chicken, fish, and tofu, are an important element of any balanced diet because they include vital amino acids that the body need to maintain muscle mass and repair tissue.

Good fats, such as those found in nuts, seeds, and avocados, are essential for heart health and lowering the risk of chronic illnesses.

What to Feed Diabetes Elderly People

It is critical for diabetic older people over the age of 50 to concentrate on meals that assist manage blood sugar levels and lower the risk of diabetes complications. These are some meals that may be included in a diabetic senior person's balanced diet:

Non-starchy foods: Non-starchy vegetables such as leafy greens, broccoli, cauliflower, and peppers are rich in fiber and low in carbs, making them an ideal option for blood sugar management.

Healthy grains, such as brown rice, quinoa, and whole wheat bread, are high in fiber, which helps manage blood sugar levels and support digestive health.

Lean proteins, such as chicken, fish, and tofu, are an important element of any balanced diet because they include vital amino acids that the body need to maintain muscle mass and repair tissue.

Good fats, such as those found in nuts, seeds, and avocados, are essential for heart health and lowering the risk of chronic illnesses.

Low-fat dairy products, such as milk, yogurt, and cheese, are a wonderful source of calcium, which is essential for bone health.

What Diabetic Elderly People Should Avoid

It is critical for diabetic senior people over the age of 50 to avoid meals that might cause blood sugar levels to jump and raise the risk of diabetes complications. Following are some examples of items to avoid or restrict in a diabetic senior person's balanced diet:

Processed foods, such as chips, cookies, and candies, are often heavy in sugar and refined carbs, causing blood sugar levels to increase.

Sugary drinks, such as soda, fruit juice, and sweetened tea, are heavy in sugar and calories and may cause blood sugar levels to jump.

Fried foods, such as french fries and fried chicken, are rich in saturated fat and calories, increasing the risk of heart disease and other chronic illnesses.

Meal Planning Suggestions

Meal preparation might be difficult for diabetes old people over the age of 50, however there are several ideas that can help:

Prepare ahead of time: Preparing ahead of time may assist to ensure that meals are balanced and suit the nutritional requirements of diabetic older people. This may also assist to lessen the likelihood of overeating or making poor dietary choices. Portion management may help diabetic senior people consume the proper quantity of food, which can help regulate blood sugar levels and avoid overeating.

Choose healthy snacks: Eating nutritious snacks like fruits, vegetables, and nuts will help keep blood sugar levels stable between meals.

Check blood sugar levels: It is critical for diabetic senior people over the age of 50 to frequently monitor their blood sugar levels, as this may assist to spot possible issues and make required changes to their diet and medication.

Drink enough of water: Drinking plenty of water may help manage blood sugar levels and avoid dehydration, which is especially essential for diabetic senior people.

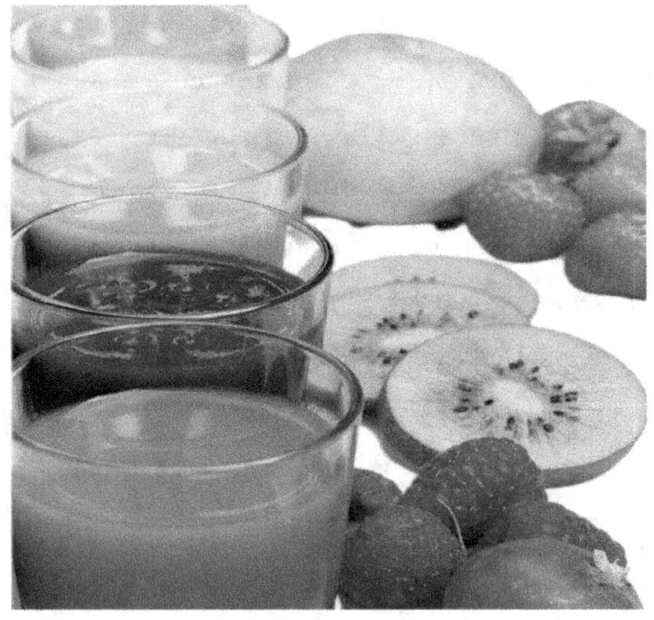

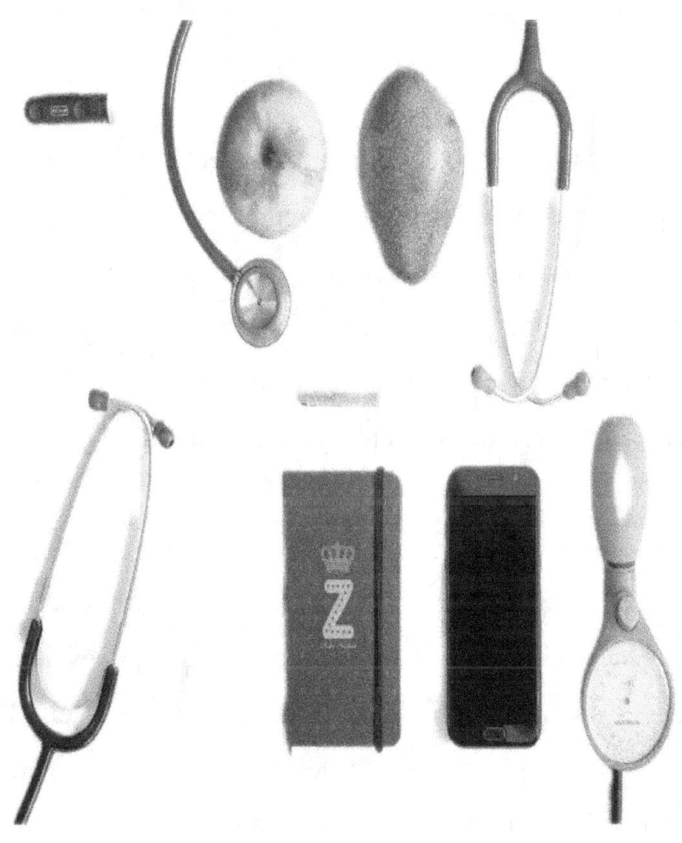

CHAPTER 3:

DIABETES COMPREHENSION

Diabetes Types

Diabetes is a chronic condition that affects millions of people worldwide. There are several types of diabetes, each with its own unique characteristics and management strategies. In this article, we will discuss the different types of diabetes that can develop after the age of 50, including their causes, symptoms, and treatment options.

Type 2 Diabetes

Type 2 diabetes is the most common form of diabetes that develops after the age of 50. This type of diabetes occurs when the body becomes resistant to insulin or does not produce enough insulin to regulate blood sugar levels. This can result in high blood sugar levels, which can cause a variety of symptoms and health complications.

Causes of Type 2 Diabetes

The exact cause of type 2 diabetes is not known, but it is believed to be caused by a combination of genetic and lifestyle factors. Some of the risk factors for type 2 diabetes include:

- **Age**: The risk of developing type 2 diabetes increases with age, particularly after the age of 50.
- **Obesity**: Being overweight or obese can increase the risk of developing type 2 diabetes, as excess body fat can interfere with insulin production and increase insulin resistance.
- **Family history:** Having a family history of diabetes can increase the risk of developing type 2 diabetes.
- **Sedentary lifestyle:** Lack of physical activity can increase the risk of developing type 2 diabetes, as exercise can help to improve insulin sensitivity and regulate blood sugar levels.
- **Unhealthy diet:** A diet high in processed foods, refined carbohydrates, and sugar can increase the risk of developing type 2 diabetes.

Symptoms of Type 2 Diabetes

The symptoms of type 2 diabetes can vary depending on the severity of the condition. Some of the common symptoms of type 2 diabetes include:

- Increased thirst and urination
- Fatigue
- Blurred vision
- Slow healing wounds
- Numbness or tingling in the hands or feet
- Recurring infections

Treatment of Type 2 Diabetes

The treatment of type 2 diabetes typically involves a combination of lifestyle modifications, medication, and regular monitoring of blood sugar levels.

Some of the treatment options for type 2 diabetes include:

Diet and exercise: A healthy diet and regular exercise can help to improve insulin sensitivity and regulate blood sugar levels.

Medication: Medications such as metformin, sulfonylureas, and insulin can help to regulate blood sugar levels and reduce the risk of complications associated with type 2 diabetes.

Blood sugar monitoring: Regular monitoring of blood sugar levels can help to identify any potential problems and make adjustments to treatment as necessary.

Gestational Diabetes

Gestational diabetes is a type of diabetes that occurs during pregnancy. This type of diabetes typically develops in the second or third trimester of pregnancy and resolves after delivery. However, women who develop gestational diabetes are at an increased risk of developing type 2 diabetes later in life.

Causes of Gestational Diabetes

The exact cause of gestational diabetes is not known, but it is believed to be caused by hormonal changes that occur during pregnancy. These hormonal changes can interfere with insulin production and increase insulin resistance, leading to high blood sugar levels.

Symptoms of Gestational Diabetes

The symptoms of gestational diabetes are similar to those of type 2 diabetes and can include:

- Increased thirst and urination
- Fatigue
- Blurred vision

- Slow healing wounds
- Numbness or tingling in the hands or feet
- Recurring infections
- Treatment of Gestational Diabetes

The treatment of gestational diabetes typically involves a combination of lifestyle modifications and regular monitoring of blood sugar levels. Some of the treatment options for gestational diabetes include:

Diet and exercise: A healthy diet and regular exercise can help to improve insulin sensitivity and regulate blood sugar levels

Blood sugar monitoring: Regular monitoring of blood sugar levels can help to identify any potential problems and make adjustments to treatment as necessary.

Medication: In some cases, medication may be needed to regulate blood sugar levels during pregnancy.

Gestational diabetes usually resolves after delivery, but women who have had gestational diabetes are at an increased risk of developing **type 2 diabetes later in life.** Therefore, it is important for women who have had gestational diabetes to maintain a healthy lifestyle and regular monitoring of their blood sugar levels.

LADA (Latent Autoimmune Diabetes in Adults)

LADA, also known as type 1.5 diabetes, is a type of diabetes that shares features of both type 1 and type 2 diabetes. It is a slowly progressive autoimmune disease that typically develops in adulthood and can be difficult to diagnose.

Causes of LADA

LADA is caused by an autoimmune response in which the body's immune system attacks and destroys the insulin-producing cells in the pancreas. This results in a gradual decrease in insulin production and an increase in blood sugar levels.

Symptoms of LADA

The symptoms of LADA are similar to those of type 2 diabetes and can include:

- Increased thirst and urination
- Fatigue
- Blurred vision

- Slow healing wounds
- Numbness or tingling in the hands or feet
- Recurring infections
- Treatment of LADA

The treatment of LADA typically involves a combination of lifestyle modifications and medication. Some of the treatment options for LADA include:

Diet and exercise: A healthy diet and regular exercise can help to improve insulin sensitivity and regulate blood sugar levels.

Blood sugar monitoring: Regular monitoring of blood sugar levels can help to identify any potential problems and make adjustments to treatment as necessary.

Medication: People with LADA may need insulin therapy to regulate blood sugar levels.

It is important for people with LADA to have regular check-ups and blood sugar monitoring to ensure that their diabetes is being managed effectively.

Diabetes's Effects on the Body

Diabetes is a chronic disease that affects how the body processes glucose, a form of sugar that serves as the body's principal energy source. Diabetes occurs when a person's body either does not create enough insulin (a hormone that helps control blood sugar levels) or does not utilise insulin efficiently.

Diabetes may have a serious influence on the body, especially in elderly people over the age of 50. In this post, we will look at the consequences of diabetes on the body beyond the age of 50.

The circulatory system

The effect of diabetes on the cardiovascular system is one of the most important effects of diabetes on the body. High blood sugar levels may cause damage to the blood vessels and nerves that regulate the heart and blood arteries, increasing the risk of heart disease and stroke. This danger is especially significant in diabetic elderly persons.

According to research, diabetic older persons are more likely to develop atherosclerosis (plaque accumulation in the arteries) and hypertension (high blood pressure), both of which are important risk factors for heart disease and stroke. Diabetes may also raise the risk of a heart attack, peripheral artery disease, and heart failure.

The Nervous System

Diabetes may potentially have serious consequences for the neurological system. Blood sugar levels that are too high may harm the nerves that govern the body's numerous systems, including the sensory and autonomic nervous systems.

As a consequence, elderly people with diabetes may have a variety of nerve-related symptoms, such as numbness or tingling in their hands and feet, weakness, and difficulties with coordination.

Diabetes may also raise the risk of diabetic neuropathy, a kind of nerve damage that can lead to significant problems including foot ulcers and infections. Diabetic neuropathy may lead to amputation in extreme circumstances.

Kidneys

Diabetes may also harm the kidneys, which are in charge of filtering waste from the blood. Excessive blood sugar levels may damage the small blood vessels in the kidneys, resulting in diabetic nephropathy. Diabetic nephropathy may progress to kidney failure, a dangerous illness that requires dialysis or a kidney transplant.

Eyes

Diabetes may also have an impact on the eyes, resulting in cataracts, glaucoma, and diabetic retinopathy. Diabetes retinopathy occurs when high blood sugar levels damage the blood vessels in the retina, the light-sensitive region of the eye. Diabetic retinopathy may cause vision loss and perhaps blindness over time.

Moreover, older persons with diabetes may be at a higher risk of acquiring other eye diseases, such as age-related macular degeneration.

Feet

Diabetes may also affect the feet, causing a variety of foot issues such as diabetic neuropathy and impaired circulation. People with diabetes may be unable to feel pain or other sensations in their feet if the nerves in their feet are destroyed, rendering them more vulnerable to accidents and infections.

Moreover, inadequate circulation may make the body's ability to fight infections and heal wounds more challenging. As a consequence, diabetic older persons may be more prone to foot ulcers, infections, and other significant foot disorders.

Mental well-being

Diabetes may also have an effect on mental health, especially in elderly people. The stress of treating a chronic ailment may result in emotions of anxiety and despair, which can have a negative influence on one's quality of life.

Also, elderly people with diabetes may be at a higher risk of cognitive deterioration and dementia. Diabetes patients are more prone than non-diabetics to have cognitive loss, including impairments with memory and reasoning abilities, according to research.

Blood sugar control and monitorin

Maintaining good blood sugar levels is essential for general health, particularly as we become older. Around the age of 50, the chance of having type 2 diabetes grows considerably, and individuals who already have diabetes must monitor and maintain blood sugar levels even more closely. This post will go over blood sugar regulation and monitoring beyond the age of 50, as well as the need of good living practices and frequent monitoring.

Healthy living practices

Keeping good living behaviors is crucial for blood sugar management and general health, particularly for individuals over 50. Here are some suggestions for good living behaviors that might aid with blood sugar control:

Having a balanced and nutritious diet is vital for controlling blood sugar levels. Consume lots of healthy foods, such as fruits and vegetables, whole grains, and lean meats. Avoid sugary and processed meals, which may cause blood sugar levels to surge.

Frequent physical activity is essential for blood sugar management and general health. Most days of the week, aim for at least 30 minutes of moderate activity, such as brisk walking or swimming.

Keeping a healthy weight: Maintaining a healthy weight may help minimize the chance of acquiring type 2 diabetes and assist people with diabetes regulate their blood sugar levels. See a healthcare expert to determine an acceptable weight target and a strategy for reaching it.

Handling stress: Since stress may raise blood sugar levels, it is important to develop healthy strategies to handle stress. Stress may be reduced with meditation, deep breathing techniques, and regular physical activity.

Obtaining adequate rest: Sleep deprivation may increase blood sugar levels to rise, therefore it is important to get enough restorative sleep each night. Strive for a minimum of 7-8 hours of sleep every night.

Monitoring of blood sugar levels

Frequent blood sugar monitoring is essential for diabetics and may be beneficial for individuals at risk of acquiring diabetes. Here are some pointers for blood sugar monitoring beyond the age of 50:

Understand goal ranges: Consult a healthcare expert about fasting and post-meal blood sugar targets. These levels may change for older folks, so knowing what is suitable for your age and health situation is critical.

A blood glucose meter is a gadget that monitors blood sugar levels from a little drop of blood. Talk with a healthcare practitioner about how often to check blood sugar levels and how to properly use a meter.

Maintaining a journal of blood sugar measurements may assist in identifying patterns and trends over time. Talk with a healthcare expert about what information to include in a log and how often it should be updated.

Recognize high and low blood sugar symptoms: High and low blood sugar may induce a variety of symptoms such as weariness, dizziness, and disorientation. Knowing these symptoms may aid in determining if blood sugar levels are too high or too low.

Frequent monitoring may assist determine when blood sugar levels are too high or too low, and lifestyle behaviors may need to be altered appropriately. Consult a healthcare provider about proper dietary, exercise, and medication changes

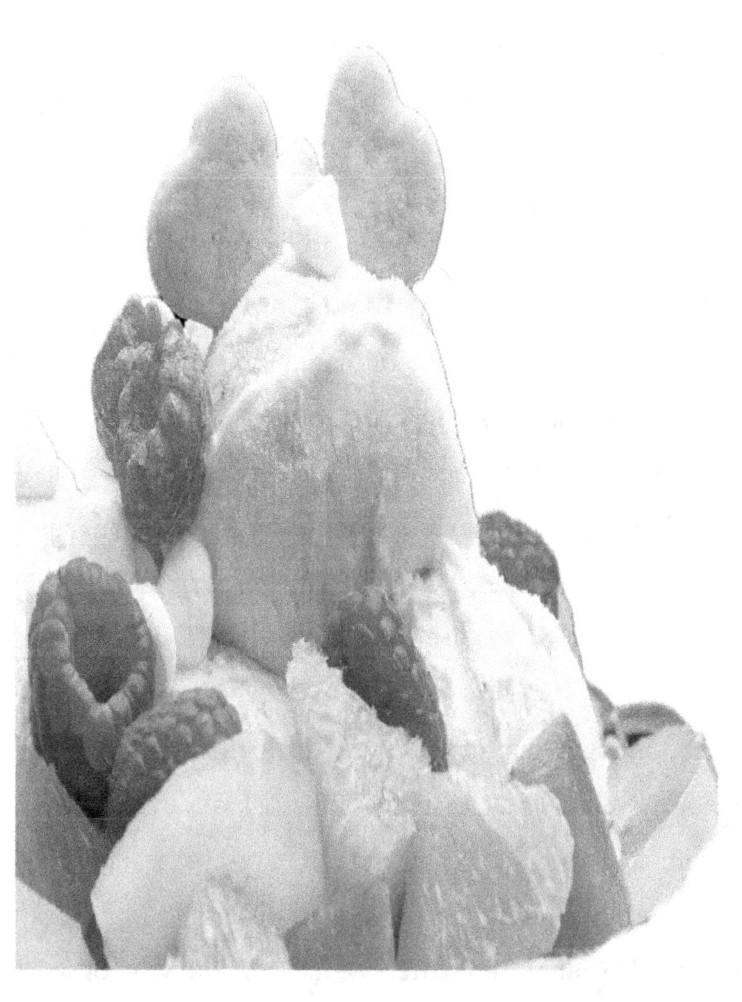

CHAPTER 4:

DIET'S ROLE IN DIABETES MANAGEMENT

The significance of a well-balanced diet

As we age, the importance of maintaining a well-balanced diet becomes increasingly critical for overall health and well-being. After the age of 50, our bodies undergo significant changes, including a decrease in muscle mass, changes in hormone levels, and a decrease in metabolic rate.

These changes can make it more difficult to maintain a healthy weight and can increase the risk of developing chronic diseases such as diabetes, heart disease, and osteoporosis. In this article, we will discuss the significance of a well-balanced diet after 50, including the importance of macronutrients, micronutrients, and hydration.

Macronutrients:Macronutrients are the nutrients that our bodies require in large amounts, including carbohydrates, proteins, and fats. Each of these macronutrients plays a unique role in our body and is critical for overall health.

Carbohydrates: Carbohydrates are the body's primary source of energy and are critical for brain function, digestion, and muscle function. However, not all carbohydrates are created equal, and it is important to focus on consuming complex carbohydrates, such as whole grains, fruits, and vegetables, rather than simple carbohydrates, such as sugary foods and drinks.

Proteins: Proteins are critical for maintaining and building muscle mass, repairing tissues, and producing hormones and enzymes. As we age, it becomes increasingly important to consume adequate amounts of protein to maintain muscle mass and prevent muscle loss. Good sources of protein include lean meats, fish, poultry, beans, and nuts.

Fats: Fats are essential for hormone production, energy production, and nutrient absorption. However, it is important to focus on consuming healthy fats, such as those found in nuts, seeds, avocados, and fatty fish, and limiting saturated and trans fats.

Micronutrients:Micronutrients are the nutrients that our bodies require in smaller amounts, including vitamins and minerals. These nutrients play critical roles in our body, including supporting immune function, bone health, and energy production.

Vitamins: Vitamins are essential for overall health and well-being and are critical for many functions in the body, including immune function, energy production, and bone health. Good sources of vitamins include fruits, vegetables, whole grains, and fortified foods.

Minerals: Minerals are essential for many bodily functions, including bone health, nerve function, and immune function. Good sources of minerals include dairy products, leafy greens, whole grains, and nuts.

Hydration:Staying hydrated is critical for overall health and well-being, especially after the age of 50. As we age, our bodies become less efficient at regulating fluid levels, making it more important to stay adequately hydrated.

Water: Water is the best source of hydration and is critical for maintaining bodily functions such as digestion, temperature regulation, and nutrient absorption. Aim for at least 8-10 glasses of water per day.

Other fluids: Other fluids, such as herbal tea, 100% fruit juice, and low-sodium broth, can also contribute to hydration.

The Benefits of a Well-Balanced Diet After 50
Maintaining a well-balanced diet after 50 can have many benefits for overall health and well-being, including:

Maintaining a healthy weight: A well-balanced diet can help maintain a healthy weight, which can help reduce the risk of developing chronic diseases such as diabetes, heart disease, and osteoporosis.

Promoting healthy aging: A well-balanced diet can help prevent age-related conditions such as cognitive decline and muscle loss.

Boosting immune function: A well-balanced diet can help boost immune function, which can help prevent illness and disease.

Reducing inflammation: A well-balanced diet can help reduce inflammation in the body, which can help prevent chronic diseases such as arthritis and heart disease.

Improving energy levels: A well-balanced diet can help improve energy levels, making it easier to stay active and maintain a healthy lifestyle.

Tips for Maintaining a Well-Balanced Diet After 50

Focus on whole, nutrient-dense foods: Whole, nutrient-dense foods such as fruits, vegetables, whole grains, lean proteins, and healthy fats should make up the bulk of your diet.

Limit processed foods: Processed foods can be high in calories, unhealthy fats, and added sugars. Limit your consumption of processed foods and focus on whole foods instead.

Eat smaller, more frequent meals: Eating smaller, more frequent meals throughout the day can help keep blood sugar levels stable and prevent overeating.

Stay hydrated: Aim for at least 8-10 glasses of water per day, and consider other hydrating fluids such as herbal tea and low-sodium broth.

Consult with a healthcare professional: If you have specific dietary needs or health concerns, it is important to consult with a healthcare professional to develop a personalized nutrition plan.

Important nutrition for diabetes management

Diabetes is a chronic disease that impairs the body's ability to handle glucose, or blood sugar. If not appropriately treated, it may lead to a variety of health concerns, particularly in individuals over the age of 50. Nutrition is important in diabetes care since it helps control blood sugar levels and avoid complications. In this post, we will cover the significance of carbs, protein, fat, fiber, vitamins, minerals, and water in diabetes treatment beyond 50.

Carbohydrates

Carbohydrates are an essential ingredient for energy generation, but diabetics must be cautious about the kinds and amounts of carbs they ingest. Carbohydrates are converted into glucose, which raises blood sugar levels. As a result, it is critical to prioritize complex carbs that are absorbed more slowly, such as whole grains, fruits, and vegetables. White bread and sugary beverages are examples of processed and refined carbs that should be avoided.

Protein

Protein is necessary for tissue growth and repair, but it also helps regulate blood sugar levels. Protein consumption may help reduce carbohydrate absorption and minimize blood sugar rises. Protein-rich foods include lean meats, fish, poultry, eggs, beans, and nuts. Nevertheless, protein sources rich in saturated fat, such as red meat, should be avoided.

Fat

While fat is a vital source of energy and aids in hormone manufacturing, some forms of fat may raise the risk of developing heart disease. Saturated and trans fats should be avoided, but good fats found in nuts, seeds, avocados, and fatty fish should be prioritized. A diet high in omega-3 fatty acids, which are found in fatty fish, may also aid enhance insulin sensitivity and decrease inflammation.

Fiber

Fiber is essential for digestive health as well as blood sugar regulation. Fiber may help decrease the absorption of carbs and reduce blood sugar rises. Whole grains, fruits, vegetables, beans, and nuts are all high in fiber. To minimize stomach pain, it is recommended to gradually increase fiber consumption.

Minerals and vitamins

Vitamins and minerals are essential for general health and may help with diabetes control. Some vitamins and minerals may aid in the improvement of insulin sensitivity and blood sugar management. Fruits, vegetables, whole grains, and lean protein sources are all good providers of vitamins and minerals.

Vitamin D is essential for bone health and immunological function, but it may also help with blood sugar management. According to certain research, persons with diabetes have lower levels of vitamin D than those who do not have diabetes. Fatty fish, eggs, and fortified meals are all good sources of vitamin D.

Magnesium is essential for bone health and may help enhance insulin sensitivity. Nuts, healthy grains, and leafy green vegetables are high in magnesium.

Hydration

Keeping hydrated is essential for general health and may help with diabetes control. Dehydration may cause blood sugar levels to increase, so drink plenty of fluids throughout the day. Water is the greatest hydration source, but other fluids such as herbal tea and low-sugar fruit juice may also help.

Diabetes Meal Planning Suggestions

To assist manage blood sugar levels, people with diabetes should concentrate on meal planning and timing. Here are some diabetic meal planning suggestions:

Reducing portion sizes may help maintain blood sugar levels and keep you from overeating.

Spread carbohydrate consumption: Eating carbs throughout the day rather than all at once will help reduce blood sugar increases.

Have regular meals: Consuming frequent meals may aid in the regulation of blood sugar levels and the prevention of overeating.

4. Emphasize whole foods: Nutrient-dense whole meals including fruits, vegetables, whole grains, and lean meats may help manage blood sugar levels.

Processed and refined foods, such as white bread and sugary beverages, should be avoided since they may induce blood sugar rises.

Good fats, such as those found in nuts, seeds, avocados, and fatty fish, may help manage blood sugar levels and increase insulin sensitivity.

Consume plenty of water throughout the day to help manage blood sugar levels and avoid dehydration.

Monitoring blood sugar levels, in addition to meal planning, is essential for diabetes control. Blood sugar monitoring may help spot patterns and make dietary and pharmaceutical modifications as required. It is critical to collaborate with a healthcare physician to develop an appropriate blood sugar monitoring routine.

Daily calorie intake recommendation

As we age, our bodies undergo various changes, including a decrease in muscle mass, which can affect our daily calorie needs. Therefore, it is essential to understand the recommended daily calorie intake for individuals over the age of 50 to maintain optimal health.

Factors Affecting Calorie Intake Recommendation after 50

Several factors can influence daily calorie intake requirements, including age, gender, height, weight, activity level, and health status.

Age: As we age, our bodies require fewer calories due to a decrease in muscle mass and metabolism. Therefore, the daily calorie intake recommendations decrease with age.

Gender: Men typically require more calories than women due to a higher muscle mass and metabolism.

Height and weight: Taller and heavier individuals require more calories to maintain their weight and meet their daily energy needs.

Activity level: Individuals who are more physically active require more calories to support their increased energy needs.

Health status: Medical conditions, such as diabetes, may require specific dietary recommendations, which can affect daily calorie intake recommendations.

Daily Calorie Intake Recommendations after 50

The daily calorie intake recommendations for individuals over the age of 50 depend on various factors, including gender, age, weight, height, and activity level. Generally, the daily calorie intake recommendations decrease as we age, due to a decrease in muscle mass and metabolism.

The United States Department of Agriculture (USDA) provides general guidelines for daily calorie intake based on age, gender, and activity level. For example, for sedentary women over 50, the USDA recommends a daily calorie intake of 1,600 to 1,800 calories, while sedentary men over 50 should consume 2,000 to 2,200 calories per day. However, these recommendations are general guidelines and may not be suitable for everyone.

It is essential to work with a healthcare provider or registered dietitian to determine an appropriate daily calorie intake recommendation based on individual factors, such as health status, activity level, and body composition.

Factors to Consider for Daily Calorie Intake Recommendations after 50

Muscle mass: As we age, our muscle mass decreases, which can affect our daily calorie needs. Therefore, it is essential to incorporate strength training exercises and adequate protein intake to maintain muscle mass and support daily calorie needs.

Health conditions: Certain health conditions, such as diabetes, may require specific dietary recommendations, which can affect daily calorie intake recommendations. It is important to work with a healthcare provider or registered dietitian to develop an individualized nutrition plan based on health status.

Activity level: Physical activity plays a critical role in daily calorie needs. Individuals who are more physically active may require more calories to support their energy needs. It is essential to incorporate regular physical activity into daily routines and adjust calorie intake accordingly.

Nutrient needs: Calorie intake should be balanced with nutrient needs. A diet rich in whole foods, including fruits, vegetables, whole grains, lean proteins, and healthy fats, can provide essential nutrients and support overall health.

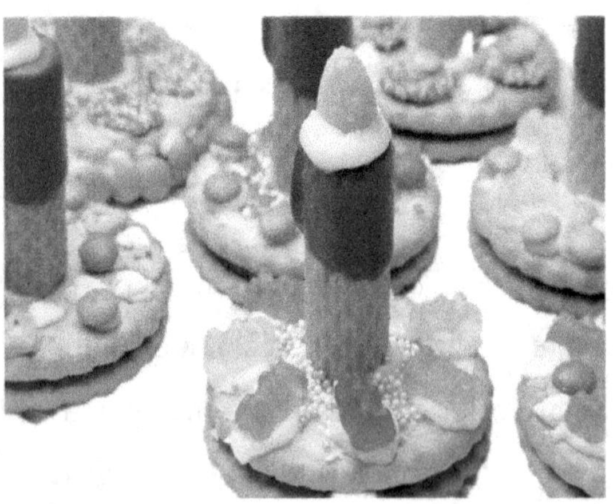

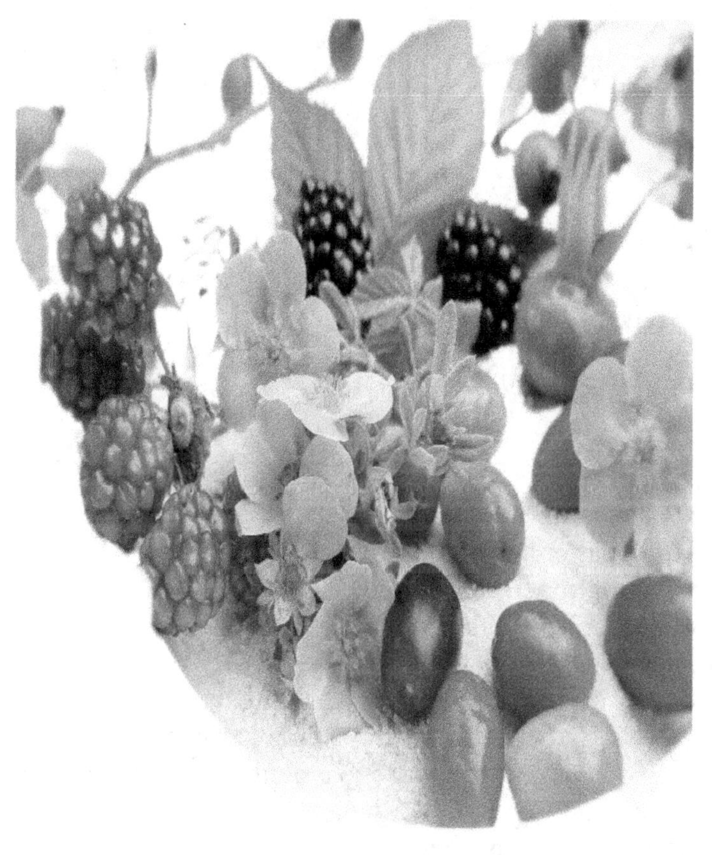

CHAPTER 5:

30 DAYS MEAL PLAN FOR DIABETIC

Day 1:

Scrambled eggs with spinach, mushrooms, and whole wheat bread for breakfast.

Ingredients:
- 2 eggs
- a quarter cup spinach
- a quarter cup mushrooms
- 1 whole wheat bread piece

Instructions:
1. Set aside the eggs after whisking them in a basin.
2. Melt butter in a nonstick pan over medium heat.
3. Cook until the spinach is wilted and the mushrooms are cooked, about 5 minutes.
4. Pour the eggs over the veggies and gently stir until the eggs are cooked through.
5. With a piece of whole wheat bread, serve.
- Preparation time: 10 minutes

Salad with grilled chicken and balsamic vinaigrette for lunch

Ingredients:
- grilled chicken breast 3 ounces
- 2 cups greens, mixed
- 1 pound cherry tomatoes
- 1/4 cup cucumber slices
- 1/4 cup red onion, sliced
- 2 tablespoons balsamic vinaigrette

Instructions:
1. Grill the chicken breast until it is thinly sliced.
2. Combine the mixed greens, cherry tomatoes, sliced cucumbers, and red onion in a large mixing basin.
3. To the bowl, add the cut chicken.
4. Toss the salad with the balsamic vinaigrette to mix.
- Preparation time: 15 minutes

Baked salmon with roasted veggies for dinner

Ingredients:
- 4 oz. fillet of salmon
- 1 cup vegetable mixture (carrots, broccoli, cauliflower)
- 1 tablespoon olive oil
- Season with salt and pepper to taste.

Instructions:
1. Preheat the oven to 375 degrees Fahrenheit.
2. Season the salmon fillet with salt and pepper and place it on a baking pan.
3. Toss the mixed veggies with olive oil, salt, and pepper in a separate bowl.

4. Arrange the veggies on the baking sheet around the fish.
5. Bake for 15-20 minutes, or until the salmon is done and the veggies are soft.
- Preparation time: 20 minutes

Day 2:

Greek yogurt with berries and almonds for breakfast

Ingredients:
- 1/2 cup plain Greek yogurt
- 1/4 cup berry mixture (strawberries, blueberries, raspberries)
- 1 tablespoon chopped nuts (almonds and walnuts)

Instructions:
1. In a mixing dish, combine the Greek yogurt and the chopped nuts.
2. Place the berries on top of the yogurt.
- Preparation time: 5 minutes
-

Tuna salad with whole wheat crackers for lunch

Ingredients:
- 1 drained can tuna in water
- 1/4 cup celery, chopped
- 1/4 cup red onion, chopped
- 2 tablespoons light mayonnaise
- Season with salt and pepper to taste.

- 5 whole grain crackers

Instructions:
1. Combine the tuna, celery, red onion, and light mayonnaise in a mixing bowl.
2. Season to taste with salt and pepper.
3. With whole wheat crackers, serve.
- Preparation time: 10 minutes

Dinner: Stir-fried beef with brown rice

Ingredients:
- 3 oz. thinly sliced sirloin of beef
- 1 cup veggies (carrots, broccoli, and bell peppers)
- 1/2 cup brown rice, cooked
- 1 tablespoon olive oil
- 1 tablespoon soy sauce (low sodium)

Instructions:
1. Over high heat, heat a nonstick skillet.
2. Cook until the sliced meat is browned on both sides.
3. Stir-fry the mixed veggies in the pan until they are tender-crisp.
4. Cook the brown rice according to package directions in a separate pot.
5. Combine the cooked brown rice with the meat and veggies in the skillet.
6. Drizzle the stir-fry with low-sodium soy sauce and whisk to mix.
- Preparation time: 25 minutes

Day 3:

Oatmeal with sliced banana and almonds for breakfast

Ingredients:
- 1/2 cup oats, old-fashioned
- 1 cup of water
- 1/2 sliced banana
- 1 tablespoon chopped nuts (almonds and walnuts)

Instructions:
1. Bring the water to a boil in a saucepan.
2. Reduce the heat to low and add the oats.
3. Cook, stirring periodically, for 5-7 minutes.
4. Serve the oats with sliced bananas and chopped nuts on top.
- Preparation time: 10 minutes

Soup with chicken and vegetables for lunch

Ingredients:
- 3 oz. shredded cooked chicken breast
- 1 cup vegetable mixture (carrots, celery, onion)
- 2 cups chicken broth (low sodium)
- Season with salt and pepper to taste.

Instructions:
1. Bring the chicken stock to a boil in a saucepan.
2. Reduce the heat to low and add the mixed veggies.
3. Cook for about 10-15 minutes, or until the veggies are soft.

4. Cook for 5 minutes more after adding the shredded chicken to the saucepan.
5. Season to taste with salt and pepper.
- Preparation time: 20 minutes

Grilled shrimp skewers with quinoa salad for dinner

Ingredients:
- 1 pound big peeled and deveined shrimp
- 1 tablespoon olive oil
- 2 minced garlic cloves
- 1 tablespoon lemon juice
- 1 teaspoon paprika
- 1/2 teaspoon cumin
- To taste, season with salt and black pepper.
- Wooden skewers that have been soaked in water for at least 30 minutes
- 1 quinoa cup
- half a cucumber, diced half a red bell pepper, diced half a red onion, diced
- 1/4 cup chopped fresh parsley
- 2 tablespoons fresh lemon juice
- 2 tablespoons olive oil
- To taste, season with salt and black pepper.

Instructions:
1. Combine the olive oil, garlic, lemon juice, paprika, cumin, salt, and black pepper in a medium mixing bowl. Toss in the shrimp to coat. Refrigerate for 30 minutes with the cover on.
2. Preheat the grill to medium-high temperature.
3. Thread the shrimp onto the skewers made of wood.

4. Grill the shrimp skewers for 2-3 minutes each side, or until well cooked and slightly browned.
5. Prepare the quinoa salad in the meanwhile. Follow the package directions for cooking the quinoa. Combine cooked quinoa, cucumber, red bell pepper, red onion, and parsley in a large mixing basin.
6. Whisk together lemon juice, olive oil, salt, and black pepper in a small bowl. Toss the quinoa salad with the dressing to blend.
7. Serve the grilled shrimp skewers beside the quinoa salad.
- Preparation time: 1 hour (including marinating)

Preparation Lunch is a turkey wrap with vegetables and hummus.

Ingredients:
- 3 oz. sliced turkey breast
- 1 whole grain wrap
- 1/4 cup mixed veggies
- 2 tablespoons hummus

Instructions:
1. On the whole wheat wrap, spread the hummus.
2. On top of the hummus, layer the sliced turkey and mixed veggies.
3. Wrap it firmly and split it in two.
- Preparation time: 10 minutes

Baked cod with roasted veggies for dinner

Ingredients:
- 4 oz. fillet of cod
- 1 cup mixed veggies (carrots, broccoli, cauliflower)

- 1 tablespoon olive oil
- Season with salt and pepper to taste.

Instructions:
1. Preheat the oven to 375 degrees Fahrenheit.
2. Line a baking sheet with parchment paper and place the fish fillet on it.
3. Season with salt and pepper to taste.
4. Toss the mixed veggies with olive oil and season with salt and pepper in a separate bowl.
5. Place the veggies on a baking sheet beside the fish.
6. Bake for 20-25 minutes, or until the fish is done and the veggies are soft.

- Preparation time: 20 minutes

Day 5:

Greek yogurt with berries and granola for breakfast

Ingredients:
- 1/2 cup Greek yogurt, plain
- 1/2 cup berries (strawberries, blueberries, and raspberries)
- 1 granola cup

Instructions:
1. In a mixing dish, combine the Greek yogurt and mixed berries.
2. Garnish with granola.

- Preparation time: 5 minutes

Tuna salad with avocado and cucumber for lunch

Ingredients:
- 3 oz. drained canned tuna
- 1/2 sliced avocado
- 1/2 sliced cucumber
- 1 tablespoon olive oil
- Season with salt and pepper to taste.

Instructions:
1. Combine the canned tuna, olive oil, and salt and pepper in a mixing bowl.
2. Serve the tuna salad with avocado and cucumber slices.
- Preparation time: 10 minutes

Dinner: Stir-fried beef and vegetables with brown rice

Ingredients:
- 3 oz. beef, thinly sliced
- 1 cup vegetable mixture (broccoli, snow peas, bell pepper)
- 1/2 cup brown rice, cooked
- 1 tablespoon soy sauce (low sodium)
- 1 tablespoon olive oil

Instructions:
1. In a pan over medium-high heat, heat the olive oil.
2. Cook until the meat is browned.
3. Cook the mixed veggies until they are tender-crisp.
4. Cook the brown rice according to package directions in a separate pot.

5. Combine the cooked brown rice with the meat and veggies in the skillet.
6. Drizzle the stir-fry with low-sodium soy sauce and whisk to mix.
● Preparation time: 25 minutes

Day 6:

Scrambled eggs with spinach and whole wheat bread for breakfast

Ingredients:
● 2 eggs
● 1/4 cup chopped spinach
● 1 whole wheat bread piece

Instructions:
1. Set aside the eggs after whisking them in a basin.
2. Melt butter in a nonstick pan over medium heat.
3. Cook until the spinach is wilted, about 5 minutes.
4. Pour the eggs over the spinach and gently stir until the eggs are cooked through.
5. With a piece of whole wheat bread, serve.
● Preparation time: 15 minutes

Soup with chicken and vegetables for lunch

Ingredients:
● 3 oz. shredded cooked chicken breast
● 1 cup vegetable mixture (carrots, celery, onion)
● 2 cups chicken broth (low sodium)

- Season with salt and pepper to taste.

Instructions:
1. Bring the chicken stock to a boil in a saucepan.
2. Reduce the heat to low and add the mixed veggies.
3. Cook for about 10-15 minutes, or until the veggies are soft.
4. Cook for 5 minutes more after adding the shredded chicken to the saucepan.
5. Season to taste with salt and pepper.
- Preparation time: 20 minutes

Salmon and roasted veggies for dinner

Ingredients:
- 4 oz. fillet of salmon
- 1 cup mixed veggies (carrots, broccoli, cauliflower)
- 1 tablespoon olive oil
- Season with salt and pepper to taste.

Instructions:
1. Preheat the oven to 375 degrees Fahrenheit.
2. Line a baking sheet with parchment paper and place the salmon fillet on it.
3. Season with salt and pepper to taste.
4. Toss the mixed veggies with olive oil and season with salt and pepper in a separate bowl.
5. Place the veggies and fish on the same baking sheet.

Bake for 20-25 minutes, or until the salmon is done and the veggies are soft.
- Preparation time: 20 minutes

Day 7:

Whole grain cereal with almond milk and banana for breakfast

Ingredients:
- 1 whole grain cereal cup
- 1/2 cup almond milk, unsweetened
- 1/2 sliced banana

Instructions:
1. Pour the whole grain cereal into a bowl.
2. Pour the almond milk on top of the cereal.
3. Serve with sliced banana on top.
- Preparation time: 5 minutes

Lunch: Whole wheat turkey and cheese sandwich with carrot sticks

Ingredients:
- 2 whole wheat bread slices
- 2 oz. turkey slices
- 1 oz. cheese slices
- 1 pound carrot sticks

Instructions:
1. Place the sliced turkey and cheese between two pieces of whole wheat bread to make the sandwich.
2. With carrot sticks on the side, serve.
- Preparation time: 10 minutes

Dinner: Stir-fried beef and broccoli with brown rice

Ingredients:
- 3 oz. beef, thinly sliced
- 1 cup florets broccoli
- 1/2 cup brown rice, cooked
- 1 tablespoon soy sauce (low sodium)
- 1 tablespoon olive oil

Instructions:
1. In a pan over medium-high heat, heat the olive oil.
2. Cook until the meat is browned.
3. Cook the broccoli florets until they are tender-crisp.
4. Cook the brown rice according to package directions in a separate pot.
5. Cooked brown rice should be added to the pan with the steak and broccoli.
6. Drizzle the stir-fry with low-sodium soy sauce and whisk to mix.
- Preparation time: 25 minutes

Day 8:

Oatmeal with apples and cinnamon for breakfast

Ingredients:
- 1/2 cup oats, old-fashioned
- 1 cup of water
- 1/2 cup almond milk, unsweetened
- 1/2 diced apple
- 1/2 teaspoon cinnamon

Instructions:
- Preparation time: 10 minutes

Lunch: omelette with spinach and feta served on whole wheat bread

Ingredients:
- 2 eggsBring the water and almond milk to a boil in a saucepan.
- Reduce the heat to low and add the old-fashioned oats.
- Simmer, stirring periodically, for 5-7 minutes, or until the oats are tender.
- Serve the oats with diced apple and cinnamon on top.
- 1/4 cup chopped spinach
- 1 oz. feta cheese crumble
- 1 whole wheat bread piece

Instructions:
1. Set aside the eggs after whisking them in a basin.
2. Melt butter in a nonstick pan over medium heat.
3. Cook until the spinach is wilted, about 5 minutes.
4. Pour the eggs over the spinach and top with feta cheese.
5. Cook, stirring occasionally, until the eggs are set and the cheese is melted.
6. With a piece of whole wheat bread, serve.
- Preparation time: 15 minutes

Baked chicken with sweet potato and green beans for dinner

Ingredients:
- 3 oz. chicken thigh
- 1 small chopped sweet potato

- 1 pound green beans
- 1 tablespoon olive oil
- Season with salt and pepper to taste.

Instructions:
1. Preheat the oven to 375 degrees Fahrenheit.
2. Drizzle olive oil over the chopped sweet potato on a baking sheet lined with parchment paper.
3. Season to taste with salt and pepper.
4. Cook for 20 minutes in the oven.
5. Season the chicken breast with salt and pepper and place it on the same baking sheet.
6. Bake for another 20-25 minutes, or until the chicken is well done.
7. Boil the green beans in a separate kettle for 5-7 minutes, or until cooked.
8. On the side, serve the chicken with sweet potato and green beans.
- Preparation time: 30 minutes

Day 9:

Greek yogurt with mixed berries and granola for breakfast

Ingredients:
- 1/2 cup Greek yogurt, plain
- 1/2 cup berries, mixed
- 1 granola cup

Instructions:
1. Scoop the Greek yogurt into a bowl.
2. Garnish with mixed berries.
3. Sprinkle with granola on top.

- Preparation time: 5 minutes

Tuna salad with whole wheat crackers for lunch

Ingredients:
- 2 oz. drained canned tuna
- 1 tbsp low-fat mayonnaise
- 1 tablespoon chopped celery
- 1 tablespoon chopped onion
- Season with salt and pepper to taste.
- 4 whole grain crackers

Instructions:
1. Combine the canned tuna, low-fat mayo, diced celery, chopped onion, salt, and pepper in a mixing dish.
2. On the side, serve with whole wheat crackers.
3. Preparation time: 10 minutes
4. Grilled pork chops with roasted asparagus for dinner

Ingredients:
- 3 oz. chops de porc
- 1/2 lb. asparagus (trimmed)
- 1 tablespoon olive oil
- Season with salt and pepper to taste.

Instructions:
1. Preheat the grill to medium-high temperature.
2. Season the pork chops with salt and pepper after brushing them with olive oil.
3. Grill the pork chops for 5-6 minutes each side, or until done.
4. Toss the asparagus in a bowl with the olive oil, salt, and pepper.
5. Roast the asparagus for 10-15 minutes at 375°F, or until tender.

6. Serve the grilled pork chops with roasted asparagus.
- Preparation time: 25 minutes

Day 10:

Scrambled eggs with whole wheat bread and orange slices for breakfast

Ingredients:
- 2 eggs
- 1 whole wheat bread piece
- 1/2 sliced orange

Instructions:
1. Set aside the eggs after whisking them in a basin.
2. Melt butter in a nonstick pan over medium heat.
3. Cook until the scrambled eggs are done.
4. Toast the whole wheat bread slice.
5. Serve the scrambled eggs with whole wheat bread and orange slices.
- Preparation time: 10 minutes

Salad with grilled chicken and balsamic vinaigrette for lunch

Ingredients:
- 3 oz. sliced grilled chicken breast
- 1 cup fresh mixed greens
- 1/4 cup halved cherry tomatoes
- 1/4 cup sliced cucumber
- 1/4 cup chopped red onion
- 1 tablespoon of balsamic vinaigrette

Instructions:

1. Place mixed greens on a platter and assemble the salad.
2. Sliced grilled chicken, cherry tomatoes, cucumber, and red onion on top.
3. Drizzle the salad with the balsamic vinaigrette.
- Preparation time: 15 minutes

Broiled fish with steamed broccoli and quinoa for dinner

Ingredients:
- 3 oz. fillet of white fish
- 1 cup florets broccoli
- 1 quinoa cup
- 1 cup of water
- 1 tablespoon olive oil
- Season with salt and pepper to taste.

Instructions:
1. Turn on the broiler to high.
2. Season the white fish fillet with salt and pepper after brushing it with olive oil.
3. Broil the fish fillet for 5-7 minutes, or until cooked through, on a broiler pan.
4. Bring the water to a boil in a separate saucepan and add the quinoa.
5. Reduce the heat to low, cover, and cook for 15-20 minutes, or until the quinoa is tender and the water has been absorbed.
6. For 5-7 minutes, steam the broccoli florets until soft.
7. Serve the broiled fish with steamed broccoli and quinoa.
- Preparation time: 30 minutes

Day 11:

Cottage cheese with sliced peaches and cinnamon for breakfast

Ingredients:
- 1 pound cottage cheese
- 1/2 sliced peach
- 1/4 teaspoon cinnamon

Instructions:
1. Scoop the cottage cheese into a bowl.
2. Serve with sliced peaches on top.
3. Sprinkle with cinnamon on top.
- Preparation time: 5 minutes

Lunch: Whole wheat pita with egg salad

Ingredients:
- 2 sliced hard-boiled eggs
- 1 tbsp low-fat mayonnaise
- 1 tablespoon chopped celery
- Season with salt and pepper to taste.
- 1 whole wheat pita, cut in half

Instructions:
1. Combine the chopped hard-boiled eggs, low-fat mayo, chopped celery, salt, and pepper in a mixing dish.
2. Fill the egg salad inside the half whole wheat pita.
- Preparation time: 15 minutes

Dinner: Stir-fried beef with brown rice

Ingredients:
- 3 oz. sliced beef sirloin

- 1 cup vegetable mixture (broccoli, bell pepper, carrot)
- 1/2 cup brown rice, cooked
- 1 tablespoon soy sauce
- 1 teaspoon sesame oil
- 1 teaspoon cornstarch
- 1 teaspoon minced garlic
- 1 teaspoon minced ginger
- Season with salt and pepper to taste.

Instructions:

1. Whisk together soy sauce, sesame oil, cornstarch, minced garlic, and minced ginger in a mixing bowl.
2. Season the beef slices with salt and pepper.
3. Over high heat, heat a nonstick skillet.
4. Stir-fry the meat in the pan for 2-3 minutes, or until browned.
5. Add the mixed veggies to the pan and cook for 3-4 minutes, or until soft.
6. Stir-fry the meat and veggies in the soy sauce mixture for 1-2 minutes, or until the sauce thickens.
7. With brown rice on the side, serve the beef stir-fry.
- Preparation time: 30 minutes

Day 12:

Oatmeal with walnuts and banana slices for breakfast

Ingredients:
- a half cup quick oats
- 1 cup of water
- 1/2 cup skim milk
- 1/4 cup walnuts, chopped

- 1/2 sliced banana

Instructions:

1. Bring the water and low-fat milk to a boil in a saucepan.
2. Add the quick oats to the saucepan and stir to combine.
3. Cook for 1-2 minutes, or until the oats are tender and the mixture has thickened.
4. Chop walnuts and slice banana on top.

- Preparation time: 10 minutes

Wrapped roasted vegetables with hummus for lunch

Ingredients:

- 1 whole grain wrap
- 1/2 cup roasted vegetable mixture (zucchini, eggplant, bell pepper)
- 2 tablespoons hummus

Instructions:

1. On the whole wheat wrap, spread hummus.
2. Serve with roasted veggies.
3. Roll up the wrap securely and cut it in two.

- Time to prepare: 25 minutes (including roasting time)

Baked salmon with roasted asparagus and sweet potato for dinner

Ingredients:

- 4 oz. fillet of salmon
- 1/2 cup spears asparagus
- 1/2 cup diced sweet potato
- 1 tablespoon olive oil
- Season with salt and pepper to taste.

Instructions:
1. Preheat the oven to 400 degrees Fahrenheit.
2. Using parchment paper, line a baking sheet.
3. Season the salmon fillet with salt and pepper and place it on the parchment paper.
4. Toss the asparagus spears and sweet potato cubes with olive oil, salt, and pepper in a separate dish.
5. Place the sweet potato and asparagus on the same baking sheet as the salmon fillet.
6. Bake for 15-20 minutes, or until the salmon is cooked through and the veggies are soft.
- Preparation time: 35 minutes

Day 13:

Greek yogurt with sliced strawberries and granola for breakfast

Ingredients:
- 1/2 cup Greek yogurt, plain
- 1/2 cup strawberries, sliced
- 1 granola cup

Instructions:
1. Scoop the plain Greek yogurt into a bowl.
2. Sprinkle with granola and cut strawberries.
- Preparation time: 5 minutes

Tuna salad lettuce wraps for lunch

Ingredients:
- 2 oz. drained canned tuna
- 1 tbsp low-fat mayonnaise

- 1/4 cup celery, chopped
- 2 hefty lettuce leaves

Instructions:

1. Combine the canned tuna, low-fat mayo, and celery in a mixing dish.
2. Sandwich the tuna salad between two lettuce leaves.
3. Wrap the tuna salad in lettuce leaves securely.

- Preparation time: 10 minutes

Turkey chili with whole wheat bread for dinner

Ingredients:

- 3 oz. turkey burgers
- 1/2 cup washed and drained canned kidney beans
- 1/2 cup chopped canned tomatoes
- 14 cup finely chopped onion
- 1 teaspoon minced garlic

Instructions

1. Cook the ground turkey in a nonstick pan until browned.
2. To the pan, add the canned kidney beans, canned diced tomatoes, chopped onion, minced garlic, chili powder, salt, and pepper.
3. Simmer for 10-15 minutes, or until all of the flavors are combined.
4. With a piece of whole wheat bread on the side, serve the turkey chili.

- Preparation time: 30 minutes

Day 14:

Veggie omelet with whole wheat bread for breakfast

Ingredients:
- 2 eggs
- 1/4 cup mixed veggies
- 1 tablespoon olive oil
- Season with salt and pepper to taste.
- 1 toasted piece whole wheat toast

Instructions:
1. Whisk the eggs with salt and pepper in a mixing dish.
2. Heat the olive oil in a nonstick skillet over medium heat.
3. Saute the mixed veggies in the pan for 2-3 minutes, or until soft.
4. Pour the whisked eggs over the veggies and simmer until the eggs are set.
5. Serve the omelet folded in half with a piece of whole wheat bread on the side.
- Preparation time: 15 minutes

Lunch: Stir-fried chicken and vegetables with brown rice

Ingredients:
- 3 oz. sliced boneless, skinless chicken breast
- 1/2 cup mixed veggies
- 1/4 cup onion, sliced
- 1 tablespoon soy sauce (low sodium)
- 1 tablespoon rice vinegar

- 1 teaspoon minced garlic
- 1 teaspoon grated ginger
- 1/2 cup brown rice, cooked

Instructions:

1. Warm a tiny quantity of olive oil in a nonstick skillet over medium heat.
2. Saute the sliced chicken breast for 3-4 minutes, or until browned.
3. To the pan, add the mixed veggies, sliced onion, chopped garlic, and grated ginger.
4. Cook for another 5-7 minutes, or until the veggies are soft.
5. Stir together the low-sodium soy sauce and rice vinegar in the skillet.
6. Serve the stir-fry chicken and vegetables over a bed of cooked brown rice.

- Preparation time: 30 minutes

Roasted turkey breast with roasted Brussels sprouts and sweet potato for dinner

Ingredients:

- 4 oz. turkey thigh
- 1/2 cup halved Brussels sprouts
- 1/2 cup diced sweet potato
- 1 tablespoon olive oil
- Season with salt and pepper to taste.

Instructions:

1. Preheat the oven to 400 degrees Fahrenheit.
2. Using parchment paper, line a baking sheet.
3. Season the turkey breast with salt and pepper and place it on the parchment paper.

4. Toss the Brussels sprouts and sweet potato cubes with olive oil, salt, and pepper in a separate dish.
5. Place the sweet potato and Brussels sprouts on the same baking sheet as the turkey breast.
6. Bake for 20-25 minutes, or until the turkey is cooked through and the veggies are soft.
- Preparation time: 35 minutes

Day 15:

Overnight oats with blueberries and almonds for breakfast

Ingredients:
- 1 pound rolled oats
- 1/2 cup almond milk, unsweetened
- 1/2 cup blueberries, fresh
- 1 tablespoon sliced almonds

Instructions:
1. Combine the rolled oats and unsweetened almond milk in a container.
2. On top, scatter the fresh blueberries and sliced almonds.
3. Refrigerate the jar for at least 24 hours.
4. Stir and serve in the morning.
- Time to prepare: 5 minutes (including overnight refrigerated).

Grilled chicken and veggie skewers with quinoa salad for lunch

Ingredients:

- 3 oz. cubed boneless, skinless chicken breast
- 1/2 cup mixed veggies
- 1 tablespoon cooked quinoa
- 1 tablespoon olive oil
- Season with salt and pepper to taste.

Instructions:
1. Heat the grill to medium-high.
2. Thread the skewers with the cubed chicken breast and mixed veggies.
3. Season the skewers with salt and pepper after brushing them with olive oil.
4. Grill the skewers for 8-10 minutes, or until the chicken is cooked through and the veggies are soft, flipping regularly.
5. Serve the grilled chicken and veggie skewers with cooked quinoa on the side.

- Preparation time: 25 minutes

Baked fish with roasted asparagus and brown rice for dinner

Ingredients:
- 4 oz. fillet of cod
- 1/2 cup spears asparagus
- 1/2 cup brown rice, cooked
- 1 tablespoon olive oil
- Season with salt and pepper to taste.

Instructions:
1. Preheat the oven to 375 degrees Fahrenheit.
2. Using parchment paper, line a baking sheet.
3. Season the fish fillet with salt and pepper and place it on the parchment paper.
4. Season the asparagus spears with salt and pepper.

5. Asparagus spears should be placed on the same baking sheet as the fish fillet.
6. Bake for 15-20 minutes, or until the fish is cooked through and the asparagus is soft.
7. Serve the baked cod with prepared brown rice on the side.
- Preparation time: 30 minutes

Day 16:

Greek yogurt with mixed berries and walnuts for breakfast

Ingredients:
- 1/2 cup Greek yogurt, plain
- 1/2 cup berries (strawberries, blueberries, and raspberries)
- 1 tablespoon chopped walnuts

Instructions:
1. Combine the plain Greek yogurt and mixed berries in a mixing dish.
2. Serve with chopped walnuts on top.
- Preparation time: 5 minutes

Wrapped turkey and avocado with carrot sticks for lunch

Ingredients:
- 2 oz. turkey breast, sliced
- 1/4 sliced avocado
- 1 whole grain tortilla
- a quarter cup carrot sticks

Instructions:
1. Lay the whole wheat tortilla out flat.
2. Place the tortilla on top of the sliced turkey breast and sliced avocado.
3. To make a wrap, roll up the tortilla.
4. Serve with carrot sticks on the side.
- Preparation time: 10 minutes

Grilled salmon with roasted veggies for dinner

Ingredients:
- 4 oz. fillet of salmon
- 1/2 cup mixed veggies (peppers, onions, mushrooms)
- 1 tablespoon olive oil
- Season with salt and pepper to taste.

Instructions:
1. Heat the grill to medium-high.
2. Season the salmon fillet with salt and pepper after brushing it with olive oil.
3. Thread the skewers with the mixed veggies.
4. Season the skewers with salt and pepper after brushing them with olive oil.
5. Grill the salmon fillet and vegetable skewers for 8-10 minutes, or until the fish is cooked through and the veggies are soft.
6. Serve the grilled salmon with roasted veggies on the side.
- Preparation time: 30 minutes

Day 17:

Breakfast: omelette with spinach and feta served with whole grain bread

Ingredients:
- 2 beaten eggs
- 1/4 cup chopped fresh spinach leaves
- 1 tablespoon feta cheese, crumbled
- 1 whole grain toast piece
- 1 tablespoon olive oil
- Season with salt and pepper to taste.

Instructions:
1. Melt butter in a nonstick pan over medium heat.
2. To the skillet, add the olive oil.
3. Pour in the beaten eggs and stir to coat the bottom of the skillet.
4. On top of the eggs, scatter the chopped spinach leaves and crumbled feta cheese.
5. Fold the omelette in half using a spatula.
6. Toast the whole grain bread and serve with the omelette.
- Preparation time: 15 minutes

Tuna salad with whole grain crackers for lunch

Ingredients:
- 2 oz. drained canned tuna
- 1/4 cup celery, chopped
- 1 tablespoon chopped onion
- 1 tablespoon Greek yogurt

- 1 tablespoon olive oil
- Season with salt and pepper to taste.
- Crackers made from whole grains

Instructions:

1. Combine the canned tuna, chopped celery, diced onion, plain Greek yogurt, olive oil, salt, and pepper in a mixing dish.
2. Serve the tuna salad with whole grain crackers on the side.

- Preparation time: 10 minutes

Baked chicken with sweet potato and green beans for dinner

Ingredients:
- 4 oz. chicken thigh
- 1 little diced sweet potato
- 1 pound green beans
- 1 tablespoon olive oil
- Season with salt and pepper to taste.

Instructions:

1. Preheat the oven to 375 degrees Fahrenheit.
2. Using parchment paper, line a baking sheet.
3. Season the chicken breast with salt & pepper and place it on the parchment paper.
4. Toss the sweet potato cubes and green beans with olive oil, salt, and pepper.
5. On the same baking sheet as the chicken breast, place the sweet potato and green beans.
6. Bake for 20-25 minutes, or until the chicken is cooked through and the sweet potato is soft.
7. Serve the cooked chicken with sweet potato and green beans on the side.

- Preparation time: 30 minutes

Day 18:

Whole grain pancakes with sugar-free syrup and sliced banana for breakfast

Ingredients:
- half a cup whole wheat flour
- 1/2 cup almond milk, unsweetened
- 1 egg
- 1 teaspoon baking powder
- 1 teaspoon vanilla extract
- 1/2 sliced banana
- Syrup without sugar

Instructions:
1. In a mixing dish, combine the whole wheat flour, unsweetened almond milk, egg, baking powder, and vanilla extract.
2. Melt butter in a nonstick pan over medium heat.
3. 1/4 cup of the pancake batter should be poured into the skillet.
4. Cook the pancake until bubbles appear on the surface, then turn and cook for another minute on the other side.
5. Repeat with the rest of the pancake batter.
6. Serve the whole grain pancakes with sliced bananas and sugar-free syrup.
- Preparation time: 15 minutes

Soup with vegetables and beans served with whole grain bread for lunch

Ingredients:
- 1/2 cup onion, chopped
- 1/2 cup carrot, chopped
- 1/2 cup celery, chopped
- 1/2 cup washed and drained canned kidney beans
- 1/2 cup chopped canned tomatoes
- 2 cups vegetable broth (low sodium)
- 1 tablespoon olive oil
- Season with salt and pepper to taste.
- 1 whole grain bread piece

Instructions:
1. In a medium-sized saucepan, heat the olive oil.
2. Saute the chopped onion, carrot, and celery in the saucepan until soft.
3. To the saucepan, add the canned kidney beans, canned chopped tomatoes, and low-sodium vegetable broth.
4. Bring the soup to a simmer and continue to boil for 10-15 minutes, or until the veggies are soft and the flavors have blended.
5. With a piece of whole grain bread, serve the vegetable and bean soup.
- Preparation time: 30 minutes

Dinner: Stir-fried beef with brown rice

Ingredients:
- 4 oz. sliced beef sirloin
- 1/2 cup bell pepper, sliced
- 1/2 cup onion, sliced
- 1/2 cup mushrooms, sliced

- 1 minced garlic clove
- 1 tablespoon olive oil
- Season with salt and pepper to taste.
- 1/2 cup brown rice, cooked

Instructions:

1. In a wok or big pan, heat the olive oil over high heat.
2. Stir-fry the cut beef sirloin in the wok until browned.
3. Stir-fry the sliced bell pepper, onion, mushrooms, and minced garlic for 3-5 minutes. Season with salt and pepper to taste.
4. Serve the beef stir-fry with cooked brown rice on the side.

- Preparation time: 20 minutes

Day 19:

Greek yogurt with mixed berries and almonds for breakfast

Ingredients:

- 1/2 cup Greek yogurt, plain
- 1/2 cup berries, mixed
- 1 tablespoon slivered almonds

Instructions:

1. Fill a bowl halfway with Greek yogurt.
2. Top with slivered almonds and assorted berries.
3. Serve the yogurt topped with berries and nuts.

- Preparation time: 5 minutes

Chicken salad with mixed greens for lunch

Ingredients:
- 4 oz. chopped cooked chicken breast
- 1 cup fresh mixed greens
- 1/4 cup cucumber, sliced
- 1/4 cup cherry tomatoes, sliced
- 1 tablespoon olive oil
- 1 tablespoon balsamic vinegar

Instructions:
1. Toss together the cooked chicken breast, mixed greens, sliced cucumber, and sliced cherry tomatoes in a mixing dish.
2. Drizzle with balsamic vinegar and olive oil.
3. Serve the chicken salad on a bed of mixed greens.
- Preparation time: 10 minutes

Baked salmon with roasted veggies for dinner

Ingredients:
- 4 oz. fillet of salmon
- 1/2 cup sweet potato dice
- 1/2 cup zucchini, diced
- 1/2 cup red onion, chopped
- 1 tablespoon olive oil
- Season with salt and pepper to taste.

Instructions:
1. Preheat the oven to 375 degrees Fahrenheit.
2. Using parchment paper, line a baking sheet.
3. Season the salmon fillet with salt and pepper and place it on the parchment paper.

4. Toss the sweet potato, zucchini, and red onion in a bowl with the olive oil, salt, and pepper.
5. Place the salmon fillet, sweet potato, zucchini, and red onion on the same baking sheet.
6. Bake for 20-25 minutes, or until the salmon is cooked through and the veggies are soft.
7. With roasted veggies, serve the baked salmon.
- Preparation time: 30 minutes

Day 20:

Veggie omelet with whole grain bread for breakfast

Ingredients:
- 1 egg
- 2 beaten egg whites
- 1/2 cup bell pepper, sliced
- 1/2 cup onion, sliced
- 1/2 cup mushrooms, sliced
- 1 tablespoon olive oil
- Season with salt and pepper to taste.
- 1 whole grain toast piece

Instructions:
1. Whisk together the egg and egg whites in a mixing basin until completely mixed.
2. In a nonstick skillet over medium heat, heat the olive oil.
3. Cook until the bell pepper, onion, and mushrooms are soft in the pan.
4. Pour the egg mixture over the veggies that have been sauteed.

5. Cook for 2-3 minutes, or until the eggs are set.
6. Slide the omelet onto a plate after folding it in half.
7. With a piece of whole grain bread, serve the vegetable omelet.
- Preparation time: 20 minutes

Wrapped turkey and avocado with carrot sticks for lunch

Ingredients:
- 2 oz. turkey breast, sliced
- 1/4 sliced avocado
- 1 whole wheat wrap
- 1 pound carrot sticks

Instructions:
1. Place the whole grain wrap on a platter flat.
2. On top of the wrap, layer the sliced turkey breast and sliced avocado.
3. Roll up the wrap securely.
4. With carrot sticks, serve the turkey and avocado wrap.
- Preparation time: 10 minutes

Lentil and vegetable stew for dinner

Ingredients:
- 1 cup lentils, cooked
- 1/2 cup finely chopped onion
- 1/2 cup celery, chopped
- 1/2 cup carrot, diced
- 1/2 cup bell pepper, chopped
- 2 minced garlic cloves
- 2 cups vegetable broth (low sodium)
- 1 tablespoon olive oil

- Season with salt and pepper to taste.

Instructions:
1. In a large saucepan over medium heat, heat the olive oil.
2. To the saucepan, add the chopped onion, celery, carrot, bell pepper, and minced garlic.
3. Saute the veggies for 5-7 minutes, or until softened.
4. Pour in the cooked lentils and vegetable broth.
5. Season to taste with salt and pepper.
6. Bring the stew to a boil and cook for 15-20 minutes, or until the veggies are soft and the flavors have combined.
7. Serve the lentil and vegetable stew over rice.
- Preparation time: 30 minutes

Day 21:

Scrambled eggs with spinach and whole grain bread for breakfast

Ingredients:
- 2 eggs
- 1 cup spinach, fresh
- 1 tablespoon olive oil
- Season with salt and pepper to taste.
- 1 whole grain toast piece

Instructions:
1. In a nonstick skillet over medium heat, heat the olive oil.
2. Saute the fresh spinach in the pan until wilted.
3. In a mixing dish, whisk together the eggs and season with salt and pepper.

4. Pour the eggs and spinach into the skillet.
5. Cook, stirring periodically, until the scrambled eggs are set.
6. With a piece of whole grain bread, serve the scrambled eggs.
- Preparation time: 15 minutes

Tuna salad with mixed greens for lunch

Ingredients:
- 2 oz. drained canned tuna
- 1 tablespoon chopped celery
- 1 tablespoon minced red onion
- 1 tablespoon chopped pickles
- 1 tablespoon Greek yogurt
- 1 teaspoon Dijon mustard
- Season with salt and pepper to taste.
- 1 cup fresh mixed greens
- 1 pound cherry tomatoes
- 1 tablespoon olive oil
- 1 tablespoon balsamic vinegar

Instructions:
1. In a mixing dish, combine the canned tuna, celery, red onion, pickles, plain Greek yogurt, Dijon mustard, salt, and pepper.
2. Toss the mixed greens and cherry tomatoes with olive oil and balsamic vinegar in a separate bowl.
3. Toss the tuna salad with the mixed greens.
- Preparation time: 15 minutes

Grilled chicken breast with roasted asparagus and quinoa for dinner

Ingredients:
- 4 oz. chicken thigh
- 1 cooked cup quinoa
- 1/2 lb. spears of asparagus
- 1 tablespoon olive oil
- Season with salt and pepper to taste.

Instructions:
1. Preheat the grill to medium-high.
2. Season both sides of the chicken breast with salt & pepper.
3. Grill the chicken breast for 5-6 minutes each side, or until done.
4. Season the asparagus spears with salt and pepper.
5. Place the asparagus on a baking sheet and roast for 10-15 minutes, or until tender, at 375°F.
6. Grilled chicken breast should be served with roasted asparagus and boiled quinoa.
- Preparation time: 30 minutes

Day 22:

Overnight oats with mixed berries for breakfast

Ingredients:
- 1/2 cup oats, old-fashioned
- 1/2 cup almond milk, unsweetened
- 1/2 cup berries, mixed
- 1 tablespoon chopped walnuts

- 1 teaspoon honey

Instructions:
1. Combine the old-fashioned oats and unsweetened almond milk in a mixing dish.
2. Mix in the mixed berries and walnuts.
3. Drizzle with honey to finish.
4. Refrigerate the bowl overnight, covered.
5. Give the oats a toss in the morning and enjoy!
- Time to prepare: 5 minutes (including overnight refrigerated).

Lunch: Stir-fried vegetables with brown rice

Ingredients:
- 1 cup brown rice, cooked
- 1 cup mixed veggies (broccoli, bell pepper, carrot, onion, etc.)
- 1 tablespoon olive oil
- 1 tablespoon soy sauce (low sodium)
- 1 minced garlic clove
- Season with salt and pepper to taste.

Instructions:
1. In a wok or big pan, heat the olive oil over medium-high heat.
2. To the wok or pan, add the mixed veggies and minced garlic.
3. Cook for 5-7 minutes, or until the veggies are tender-crisp.
4. Add the cooked brown rice and low-sodium soy sauce to the wok or pan.
5. Toss everything together and season to taste with salt and pepper.

6. With brown rice, serve the veggie stir-fry.
● Preparation time: 20 minutes

Baked salmon with roasted sweet potatoes and green beans for dinner

Ingredients:
● 4 oz. fillet of salmon
● 1 medium peeled and sliced sweet potato
● 1/2 lb. green beans, fresh
● 1 tablespoon olive oil
● Season with salt and pepper to taste.

Instructions:
1. Preheat the oven to 375 degrees Fahrenheit.
2. Season the salmon fillet with salt and pepper and place it on a baking pan.
3. Toss the sweet potato cubes and green beans with olive oil, salt, and pepper.
4. On a separate baking sheet, place the sweet potato and green beans.
5. Bake the salmon and veggies for 15-20 minutes, or until the fish is done and the vegetables are soft.
6. Baked salmon goes well with roasted sweet potatoes and green beans.
● Preparation time: 30 minutes

Day 23:

Greek yogurt with mixed berries and granola for breakfast

Ingredients:

- 1 cup Greek yogurt, plain
- 1/2 cup berries, mixed
- 1 granola cup

Instructions:
1. Spoon the Greek yogurt into a bowl.
2. Top with granola and mixed berries.
3. Serve and have fun!
- Preparation time: 5 minutes

Wrapped turkey and avocado with baby carrots for lunch

Ingredients:
- 2 oz. turkey breast, sliced
- 1/4 sliced avocado
- 1 whole wheat tortilla
- a quarter cup baby carrots

Instructions:
1. Place the whole grain tortilla on a platter flat.
2. Layer the tortilla with the sliced turkey breast and avocado.
3. Tuck in the edges of the tortilla as you roll it up.
4. With tiny carrots, serve the turkey and avocado wrap.
- Preparation time: 10 minutes

Dinner: Stir-fried beef and vegetables with brown rice

Ingredients:
- 4 oz. sliced beef sirloin
- 1 cup mixed veggies (broccoli, bell pepper, carrot, onion, etc.)
- 1 tablespoon olive oil

- 1 tablespoon soy sauce (low sodium)
- 1 minced garlic clove
- Season with salt and pepper to taste.
- 1 cup brown rice, cooked

Instructions:

1. In a wok or big pan, heat the olive oil over medium-high heat.
2. To the wok or pan, add the cut meat and minced garlic.
3. 3. Cook for 3-4 minutes, or until the meat is browned on both sides.

4. Stir-fry the mixed veggies in the wok or pan for another 3-4 minutes, or until the vegetables are tender-crisp.
5. Season with salt and pepper to taste after adding the low-sodium soy sauce.
6. Cooked brown rice should be served with the steak and veggie stir-fry.

- Preparation time: 20 minutes

Day 24:

Scrambled eggs with whole wheat bread and orange slices for breakfast

Ingredients:
- two huge eggs
- 1 whole wheat bread slice
- 1 medium peeled and sliced orange
- 1 tablespoon olive oil
- Season with salt and pepper to taste.

Instructions:

1. Set aside the toasted whole wheat bread.
2. Heat the olive oil in a nonstick skillet over medium heat.
3. In a mixing dish, whisk together the eggs and season with salt and pepper.
4. Scramble the eggs in the skillet until they are fully cooked.
5. Serve the scrambled eggs with whole wheat bread and slices of orange.
- Preparation time: 10 minutes

Tuna salad with mixed vegetables and whole wheat crackers for lunch

Ingredients:
- 2 oz. drained canned tuna
- 1 tablespoon light mayonnaise
- 1 teaspoon Dijon mustard
- 1/4 cup celery, chopped
- 1/4 cup onion, chopped
- 2 cups greens, mixed
- 4 whole grain crackers

Instructions:
1. Combine the canned tuna, low-fat mayonnaise, Dijon mustard, chopped celery, and diced onion in a mixing dish.
2. Place the tuna salad on top of the mixed greens on a platter.
3. With whole wheat crackers, serve the tuna salad.
- Preparation time: 10 minutes

Roasted chicken with quinoa and roasted veggies for dinner

Ingredients:
- 4 oz. chicken breast, skinless and boneless
- 1 quinoa cup
- 1 cup mixed veggies (zucchini, bell pepper, onion, etc.)
- 1 tablespoon olive oil
- Season with salt and pepper to taste.

Instructions:
1. Preheat the oven to 375 degrees Fahrenheit.
2. Season the chicken breast with salt and pepper and place it on a baking pan.
3. Roast the chicken for 25-30 minutes, or until cooked through.
4. Cook the quinoa according to package directions while the chicken roasts.
5. Toss the veggies in a bowl with olive oil, salt, and pepper.
6. Place the veggies on a separate baking sheet and roast for 15-20 minutes, or until soft.
7. With quinoa and roasted veggies, serve the roasted chicken.
- Preparation time: 40 minutes

Day 25:

Veggie omelette with whole wheat bread and grapefruit slices for breakfast

Ingredients:
- two huge eggs

- 1/4 cup mixed veggies (spinach, mushrooms, and bell pepper, for example)
- 1 whole wheat bread slice
- 1/2 peeled and sliced grapefruit
- 1 tablespoon olive oil
- Season with salt and pepper to taste.

Instructions:

1. Set aside the toasted whole wheat bread.
2. Heat the olive oil in a nonstick skillet over medium heat.
3. Saute the mixed veggies in the pan for 3-4 minutes, or until soft.
4. In a mixing dish, whisk together the eggs and season with salt and pepper.
5. Cook until the eggs are set over the veggies in the pan.
6. Fold the omelette in half and set it aside on a platter.
7. With whole wheat bread and grapefruit pieces, serve the vegetable omelette.

- Preparation time: 15 minutes

Chicken salad with whole grain crackers for lunch

Ingredients:
- 2 oz. shredded cooked chicken breast
- 1/4 cup celery, chopped
- 1/4 cup apple, chopped
- 2 tbsp plain low-fat yogurt
- 2 tablespoons low-fat mayonnaise
- 1 teaspoon Dijon mustard
- Season with salt and pepper to taste.
- 4 whole wheat crackers

Instructions:

1. In a mixing dish, combine the cooked chicken breast, celery, apple, low-fat plain yogurt, mayonnaise, Dijon mustard, salt, and pepper.
2. With whole grain crackers, serve the chicken salad.
- Preparation time: 10 minutes

Grilled salmon with brown rice and steamed broccoli for dinner

Ingredients:
- 4 oz. fillet of salmon
- 1 pound brown rice
- 1 cup florets broccoli
- 1 tablespoon olive oil
- Season with salt and pepper to taste.

Instructions:
1. Brown rice should be cooked according to package directions.
2. Preheat a grill pan to medium-high.
3. Season the salmon fillet with salt and pepper after brushing it with olive oil.
4. Grill the salmon fillet for 3-4 minutes each side, or until done.
5. Broccoli florets should be steamed until soft.
6. Grilled salmon should be served with brown rice and steamed broccoli.
- Preparation time: 30 minutes

Day 26:

Breakfast: blueberry whole wheat pancakes with scrambled eggs

Ingredients:
- half a cup whole wheat flour
- 1 teaspoon baking powder
- 1/4 teaspoon salt
- 1/2 cup skim milk
- 1 big egg
- 1/2 cup blueberries, fresh
- two huge eggs
- 1 tablespoon olive oil
- Season with salt and pepper to taste.

Instructions:
1. In a mixing dish, combine the whole wheat flour, baking powder, and salt.
2. Whisk together the low-fat milk and egg in a mixing bowl until smooth.
3. Incorporate the fresh blueberries.
4. Melt butter in a nonstick pan over medium heat.
5. Pour the pancake batter into the skillet and cook for 2-3 minutes each side, or until golden brown.
6. Heat the olive oil in a separate nonstick pan over medium heat.
7. In a mixing dish, whisk together the eggs and season with salt and pepper.
8. Scramble the eggs in the skillet until they are fully cooked.
9. Serve the blueberries and scrambled eggs on whole wheat pancakes.
- Preparation time: 20 minutes

Wrapped turkey and avocado with carrot sticks for lunch

Ingredients:
- 2 oz. turkey breast deli
- 1/4 sliced avocado
- 1 whole grain tortilla
- 1/4 cup lettuce, shredded
- 1/4 cup carrot shredded
- 1 tablespoon light mayonnaise
- Season with salt and pepper to taste.
- 1 pound carrot sticks

Instructions:
1. Spread the low-fat mayonnaise over the whole wheat tortilla.
2. To the tortilla, add the deli turkey breast, sliced avocado, shredded lettuce, shredded carrot, salt, and pepper.
3. Roll the tortilla into a tight coil.
4. With carrot sticks, serve the turkey and avocado wrap.
- Preparation time: 10 minutes

Beef and barley stew with various veggies for dinner

Ingredients:
- 4oz. beef stew meat that is lean
- a quarter cup barley
- 1/2 chopped onion
- 2 minced garlic cloves
- 2 cups beef broth (low sodium)
- 1 cup vegetable mixture (carrots, green beans, corn)
- 1 tablespoon olive oil

- Season with salt and pepper to taste.

Instructions:

1. Warm the olive oil in a big saucepan over medium heat.
2. Saute the chopped onion and minced garlic for 2-3 minutes, or until softened.
3. Cook until the beef stew meat is browned on both sides.
4. Pour in the barley and beef broth.
5. Bring the mixture to a boil, then lower to a low heat and continue to cook for 45 minutes to an hour, or until the meat and barley are cooked.
6. Cook for a further 10-15 minutes, or until the veggies are soft, in the saucepan with the mixed vegetables.
7. Season to taste with salt and pepper.
8. Serve the beef and barley stew with a variety of veggies.

- Preparation time: 1 hour

Day 27:

Greek yogurt parfait with granola and berries for breakfast

Ingredients:

- 1/2 cup Greek yogurt, plain
- 1 granola cup
- 1/2 cup berries (strawberries, blueberries, and raspberries)

Instructions:

1. Layer the plain Greek yogurt, granola, and mixed berries in a dish or cup.

2. Serve with granola and berries on top of the Greek yogurt parfait.
- Preparation time: 5 minutes

Tuna salad lettuce wraps with tomato slices for lunch

Ingredients:
- 2 oz. drained canned tuna
- 1/4 cup celery, chopped
- 1 tablespoon light mayonnaise
- 1 teaspoon Dijon mustard
- Season with salt and pepper to taste.
- 2 hefty lettuce leaves
- 2 tomato slices

Instructions:
1. In a mixing dish, combine the canned tuna, celery, low-fat mayonnaise, Dijon mustard, salt, and pepper.
2. Lay the lettuce leaves flat and top with a piece of tomato.
3. Serve the tuna salad on lettuce leaves.
4. Make lettuce wraps by firmly rolling the lettuce leaves.
5. Serve the lettuce wraps with tuna salad and tomato slices.
- Preparation time: 10 minutes

Baked chicken with sweet potato wedges and roasted Brussels sprouts for dinner

Ingredients:
- 4 oz. chicken breast, boneless and skinless

- 1 small sweet potato, peeled and cut into wedges
- 1 cup halved Brussels sprouts
- 1 tablespoon olive oil
- Season with salt and pepper to taste.

Instructions:

1. Preheat the oven to 400 degrees Fahrenheit.
2. Place the chicken breast in a baking dish and season with salt and pepper.
3. Wrap the chicken breast with sweet potato wedges and halved Brussels sprouts.
4. Dress the chicken breast, sweet potato wedges, and Brussels sprouts with the olive oil.
5. Season with salt and pepper as desired.
6. Bake for 25-30 minutes, or until the chicken is done and the sweet potato wedges and Brussels sprouts are soft.
7. Serve the cooked chicken with roasted Brussels sprouts and sweet potato wedges.

- Preparation time: 40 minutes

Day 28:

Veggie frittata with whole wheat bread and orange slices for breakfast

Ingredients:

- two huge eggs
- 2 beaten egg whites
- 14 cup finely chopped onion
- 14 cup diced bell pepper
- 1/4 cup mushrooms, sliced
- 1/4 cup spinach, chopped

- 1 tablespoon olive oil
- Season with salt and pepper to taste.
- 1 whole wheat bread piece
- 1 medium sliced orange

Instructions:

1. Preheat the oven to 375 degrees Fahrenheit.
2. Whisk together the eggs and egg whites in a mixing bowl.
3. Warm the olive oil in a nonstick oven-safe skillet over medium heat.
4. Saute the onion, bell pepper, and sliced mushrooms for 2-3 minutes, or until softened.
5. Cook for a further 1-2 minutes, or until the spinach has wilted, in the skillet.
6. Pour in the egg mixture and cook for 2-3 minutes, or until the edges begin to firm.
7. Place the pan in the oven for 10-15 minutes, or until the frittata is cooked through.
8. Toast the whole wheat bread and serve with orange slices beside the frittata.

- Preparation time: 25 minutes

Lentil and vegetable soup with whole wheat crackers for lunch

Ingredients:
- 1 pound lentils
- 1/2 chopped onion
- 2 minced garlic cloves
- 2 cups vegetable broth (low sodium)
- 1 cup vegetable mixture (carrots, green beans, corn)
- 1 tablespoon olive oil
- Season with salt and pepper to taste.

- 4 whole grain crackers

Instructions:
1. Warm the olive oil in a big saucepan over medium heat.
2. Saute the chopped onion and minced garlic for 2-3 minutes, or until softened.
3. Pour in the lentils and vegetable broth.
4. Bring the mixture to a boil, then lower to a low heat and continue to cook for 20-30 minutes, or until the lentils are cooked.
5. Cook for a further 10-15 minutes, or until the veggies are soft, in the saucepan with the mixed vegetables.
6. Season to taste with salt and pepper.
7. With whole wheat crackers, serve the lentil and vegetable soup.

- Preparation time: 45 minutes

Grilled salmon with quinoa and roasted asparagus for dinner

Ingredients:
- 4 oz. fillet of salmon
- 1 cooked cup quinoa
- 8 asparagus spears
- 1 tablespoon olive oil
- Season with salt and pepper to taste.

Instructions:
1. Preheat the grill to medium-high temperature.
2. Season both sides of the salmon fillet with salt and pepper.
3. Grill the salmon fillets for 3-4 minutes each side, or until cooked through.

4. Toss the asparagus with olive oil and season with salt and pepper while the fish cooks.
5. Place the asparagus on a baking sheet and roast for 10-15 minutes, or until tender, at 400°F.
6. Grilled salmon should be served with cooked quinoa and roasted asparagus.
* Preparation time: 30 minutes

Day 29:

Oatmeal with banana slices and walnuts for breakfast

Ingredients:
* 1 pound rolled oats
* 1 cup of water
* 1/2 sliced banana
* 1 tablespoon chopped walnuts
* 1 tablespoon honey (optional)

Instructions:
1. Bring the water to a boil in a small saucepan.
2. Reduce the heat to low and add the rolled oats to the saucepan.
3. Cook, stirring periodically, for 5-7 minutes, or until the oats are soft and the water has been absorbed.
4. Remove the saucepan from the heat and toss in the banana slices and walnuts.
5. Drizzle honey over the oats if desired.
6. Serve immediately.
* Preparation time: 10 minutes

Apple slices with almond butter as a snack

Ingredients:
- 1 medium sliced apple
- 1 tablespoon almond butter

Instructions:
1. Wash and cut the apple into wedges.
2. On each apple slice, spread almond butter.
3. As a snack, serve.
- Preparation time: 5 minutes

Tuna salad with whole wheat pita for lunch

Ingredients:
- 1 drained can tuna
- 1/4 chopped onion
- 1 celery stalk, chopped
- 1 tablespoon lemon juice
- 1 tablespoon light mayonnaise
- Season with salt and pepper to taste.
- 1 whole wheat pita, halved
- 1 cup fresh mixed greens

Instructions:
1. In a mixing dish, combine the drained tuna, diced onion, and chopped celery.
2. Combine the lemon juice and low-fat mayonnaise in a mixing dish.
3. Season to taste with salt and pepper.
4. Fill the whole wheat pita halves with the tuna salad.
5. Serve with mixed greens on the side.
- Preparation time: 15 minutes

Grilled chicken with sweet potato and green beans for dinner

Ingredients:
- 4 oz. chicken thigh
- 1 small chopped sweet potato
- 1 pound green beans
- 1 tablespoon olive oil
- Season with salt and pepper to taste.

Instructions:
1. Preheat the grill to medium-high temperature.
2. Season both sides of the chicken breast with salt & pepper.
3. Grill the chicken breasts for 4-5 minutes each side, or until cooked through.
4. While the chicken is cooking, season the sweet potato slices and green beans with salt and pepper.
5. Place the sweet potato slices and green beans on a baking sheet and roast for 15-20 minutes, or until cooked, at 400°F.
6. Grilled chicken should be served with roasted sweet potato slices and green beans.
- Preparation time: 30 minutes

Day 30:

Greek yogurt with berries and granola for breakfast

Ingredients:
- 1/2 cup Greek yogurt, nonfat
- 1/2 cup blueberries, raspberries, and strawberries

- 1/4 cup granola (low-sugar)

Instructions:

1. Fill a bowl halfway with Greek yogurt.
2. Fill the basin with the mixed berries.
3. Sprinkle with the low-sugar granola.
4. Serve chilled.

- Preparation time: 5 minutes

Carrots with hummus as a snack

Ingredients:

- 1 cup carrots, baby
- 2 tablespoons hummus

Instructions:

1. Arrange the tiny carrots on a platter after washing them.
2. Fill a small bowl halfway with hummus.
3. Using a fork, dip the small carrots into the hummus.
4. As a snack, serve.

- Preparation time: 5 minutes

Lunch consists of an egg salad sandwich with a side salad.

Ingredients:

- 2 sliced hard-boiled eggs
- 1 tablespoon light mayonnaise
- 1/4 chopped onion
- Season with salt and pepper to taste.
- 2 whole wheat bread slices
- 1 cup fresh mixed greens
- 1 tablespoon of balsamic vinaigrette

Instructions:

1. Combine the chopped hard-boiled eggs, low-fat mayonnaise, and chopped onion in a mixing dish.
2. Season to taste with salt and pepper.
3. Toast the pieces of whole wheat bread.
4. Spread the egg salad on one piece of bread and cover with the other.
5. Serve with a side salad of mixed greens dressed with balsamic vinaigrette.
- Preparation time: 15 minutes

Baked salmon with quinoa and roasted asparagus for dinner

Ingredients:
- 4 oz. fillet of salmon
- 1 quinoa cup
- 1 cup of water
- 1 asparagus bunch, trimmed
- 1 tablespoon olive oil
- Season with salt and pepper to taste.

Instructions:
1. Preheat the oven to 375 degrees Fahrenheit.
2. Season the salmon fillet with salt and pepper and place it on a baking pan.
3. Bake the salmon for 10-12 minutes, or until cooked through.
4. Rinse the quinoa and set it in a pot with 1 cup of water while the salmon cooks.
5. Bring the quinoa to a boil, then lower to a low heat and continue to cook for 15 minutes.
6. Season the trimmed asparagus with salt and pepper and toss with olive oil.

7. Place the asparagus on a baking sheet and roast for 10-12 minutes, or until tender, at 375°F.
8. Serve the baked salmon with quinoa and roasted asparagus on the side.
● Preparation time: 30 minutes

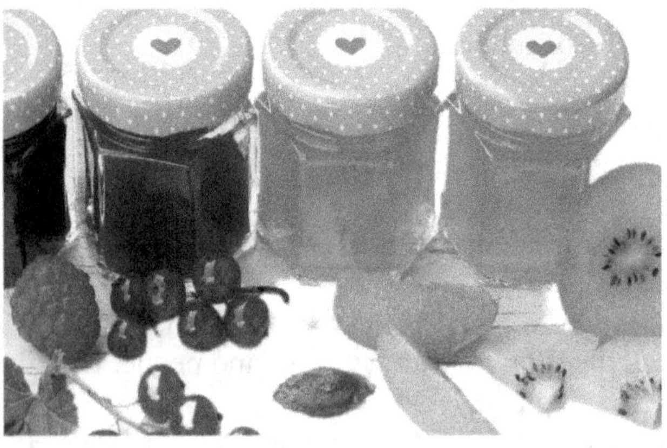

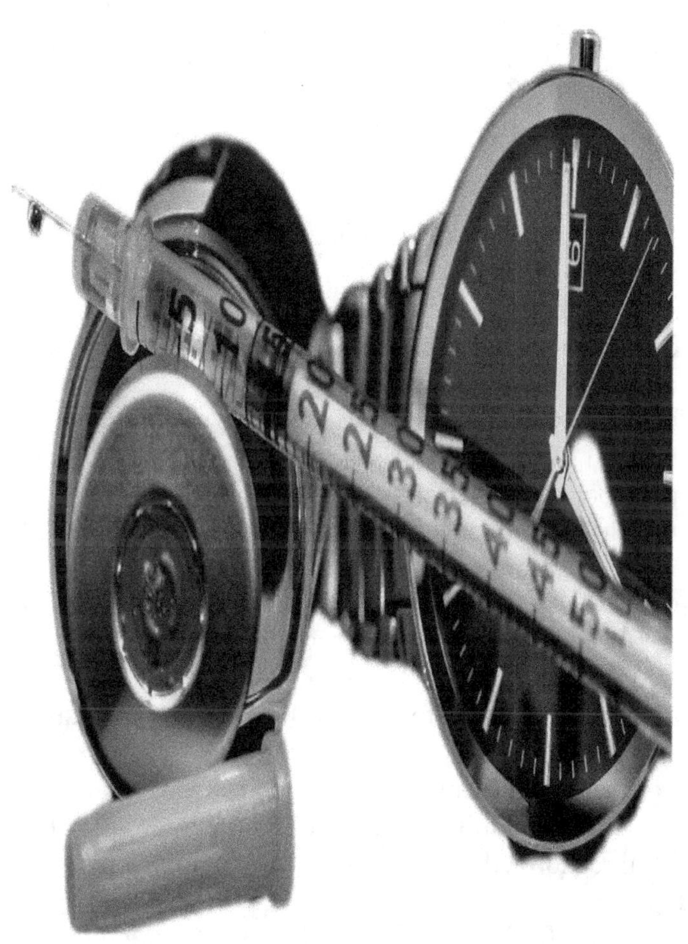

CHAPTER 6:

30 SOUPS AND STEWS RECIPE

Traditional Chicken Noodle Soup

Ingredients:
- 1 pound skinless boneless chicken breasts
- 8 cup chicken stock
- 2 servings egg noodles
- 1 cup carrots, chopped
- 1 cup celery, chopped
- 1 medium sliced onion
- 3 minced garlic cloves
- 1 teaspoon thyme dried
- 1 tsp. dried oregano
- Season with salt and black pepper to taste.

Instructions:
1. Heat the chicken stock in a large saucepan until it begins to boil.
2. Cook for 20-25 minutes, or until the chicken breasts are cooked through.
3. Take the chicken out of the pot and shred it.
4. Cook for 10-15 minutes, or until the veggies are soft, with the chopped vegetables, garlic, thyme, and oregano.
5. Cook for a further 10-12 minutes after adding the shredded chicken and egg noodles to the saucepan.
6. Season to taste with salt and black pepper.
- Preparation time: 50 minutes

Tomato Soup with Cream

Ingredients:
- 2 tbsp of olive oil
- 1 chopped onion
- 2 minced garlic cloves
- 2 cans crushed tomatoes (28 oz. each)
- 2 cup chicken stock
- 1 tsp. dried basil
- 1 tsp. dried oregano
- 1 quart thick cream
- Season with salt and black pepper to taste.

Instructions:
1. Warm the olive oil in a big saucepan over medium heat.
2. Cook for 5-7 minutes, or until the onion is transparent, with the chopped onion and garlic.
3. Bring the crushed tomatoes, chicken broth, basil, and oregano to a boil in a saucepan.
4. Reduce the heat to low and continue to cook for 15-20 minutes.
5. Puree the soup with an immersion blender until smooth.
6. Season with salt and black pepper to taste after adding the heavy cream.
- Preparation time: 50 minutes

Stew with Beef

Ingredients:
- 2 lbs beef stew meat, chopped into 1-inch cubes
- 1 tablespoon all-purpose flour
- 2 tbsp of olive oil
- 2 cups beef stock

- 1 quart red wine
- two tbsp tomato paste
- 4 minced garlic cloves
- 1 teaspoon thyme dried
- 4 peeled and sliced carrots
- 2 chopped onions
- 3 peeled and sliced potatoes
- Season with salt and black pepper to taste.

Instructions:

1. Toss the beef stew meat with the flour in a large mixing basin until evenly covered.
2. Warm the olive oil in a large saucepan over medium-high heat.
3. Cook for 5-7 minutes, or until the beef stew meat is browned on both sides.
4. Bring the beef broth, red wine, tomato paste, garlic, and thyme to a boil in a saucepan.
5. Reduce the heat to low and continue to cook for 1 hour.
6. Cook for a further 30-40 minutes, or until the veggies are soft, in the saucepan with the chopped vegetables.
7. Season to taste with salt and black pepper.
- Preparation time: 50 minutes

Soup with Lentils

Ingredients:
- 1 tablespoon extra virgin olive oil
- 1 chopped onion
- 2 minced garlic cloves
- 1 cup washed and drained dry lentils
- 4 cup chicken stock

- 2 cups kale, chopped
- 1 teaspoon thyme dried
- 1/2 teaspoon cumin powder
- Black pepper with salt
- season with pepper to taste

Instructions:

1. Warm the olive oil in a big saucepan over medium heat.
2. Cook for 5-7 minutes, or until the onion is transparent, with the chopped onion and garlic.
3. Bring the dry lentils, chicken broth, kale, thyme, and cumin to a boil in a saucepan.
4. Reduce to a low heat and cook for 30-40 minutes, or until the lentils are cooked.
5. Season to taste with salt and black pepper.

- Preparation time: 50 minutes

Soup Minestrone

Ingredients:

- 2 tbsp of olive oil
- 1 chopped onion
- 2 minced garlic cloves
- 1 can chopped tomatoes (28 oz.)
- 4 cup chicken stock
- 2 peeled and sliced carrots
- 2 celery stalks, chopped
- 1 sliced zucchini
- 1 can (15 ounces) washed and drained cannellini beans
- 1 cup tiny pasta (elbow or ditalini)
- 1 tsp. dried basil
- 1 tsp. dried oregano
- Season with salt and black pepper to taste.

Instructions:
1. Warm the olive oil in a big saucepan over medium heat.
2. Cook for 5-7 minutes, or until the onion is transparent, with the chopped onion and garlic.
3. Bring to a boil the diced tomatoes, chicken stock, chopped veggies, cannellini beans, pasta, basil, and oregano.
4. Reduce the heat to low and continue to cook for 15-20 minutes, or until the veggies are soft and the pasta is tender.
5. Season to taste with salt and black pepper.
- Preparation time: 50 minutes

Potato Soup with Cream

Ingredients:
- 4 tbsp unsweetened butter
- 1 chopped onion
- 2 minced garlic cloves
- 4 cup chicken stock
- 4 cups potatoes, peeled and diced
- 1 quart thick cream
- 1 teaspoon thyme dried
- Season with salt and black pepper to taste.

Instructions:
1. Melt the butter in a big saucepan over medium heat.
2. Cook for 5-7 minutes, or until the onion is transparent, with the chopped onion and garlic.
3. Bring the chicken stock and chopped potatoes to a boil in the saucepan.
4. Reduce to a low heat and cook for 20-25 minutes, or until the potatoes are cooked.

5. Puree the soup with an immersion blender until smooth.
6. Season with salt and black pepper to taste after adding the heavy cream and thyme.
- Preparation time: 50 minutes

Chili Vegetarian

Ingredients:
- 2 tbsp of olive oil
- 1 chopped onion
- 2 minced garlic cloves
- 1 can chopped tomatoes (28 oz.)
- 2 cups veggie broth
- 1 cup washed and drained quinoa
- two tbsp chili powder
- 1 teaspoon cumin powder
- 1 can (15 ounces) rinsed and drained black beans
- 1 can (15 ounces) washed and drained kidney beans
- Season with salt and black pepper to taste.

Instructions:
1. Warm the olive oil in a big saucepan over medium heat.
2. Cook for 5-7 minutes, or until the onion is transparent, with the chopped onion and garlic.
3. Bring the chopped tomatoes, vegetable broth, quinoa, chili powder, and cumin to a boil in a saucepan.
4. Reduce the heat to low and cook for 20-25 minutes, or until the quinoa is tender.
5. Add the black beans and kidney beans to the saucepan and cook for 5-10 minutes, or until cooked through.
6. 6. Season to taste with salt and black pepper.
- Preparation time: 50 minutes

Stew with Beef

Ingredients:
- 2 tbsp of olive oil
- 1 chopped onion
- 2 minced garlic cloves
- 2 pounds stew beef, sliced into bite-size pieces
- 4 cups beef stock
- 2 peeled and sliced carrots
- 2 celery stalks, chopped
- 2 peeled and sliced potatoes
- 1 teaspoon thyme dried
- 1 teaspoon rosemary dried
- Season with salt and black pepper to taste.

Instructions:
1. Warm the olive oil in a big saucepan over medium heat.
2. Cook for 5-7 minutes, or until the onion is transparent, with the chopped onion and garlic.
3. Brown the beef stew meat on both sides in the saucepan.
4. Bring the beef stock, chopped veggies, thyme, and rosemary to a boil in a saucepan.
5. Reduce the heat to low and continue to cook for 2-3 hours, or until the meat is tender.
6. Season to taste with salt and black pepper.
- Preparation time: 50 minutes

Tomato Soup with Cream

Ingredients:
- 2 tbsp unsweetened butter
- 1 chopped onion
- 2 minced garlic cloves

- 2 cans whole peeled tomatoes (28 oz. each)
- 2 cup chicken stock
- 1 quart thick cream
- 1 tsp. dried basil
- Season with salt and black pepper to taste.

Instructions:

1. Melt the butter in a big saucepan over medium heat.
2. Cook for 5-7 minutes, or until the onion is transparent, with the chopped onion and garlic.
3. Bring the entire peeled tomatoes (with juice) and chicken stock to a boil in a saucepan.
4. Reduce to a low heat and cook for 20-25 minutes, or until the tomatoes are soft.
5. Puree the soup with an immersion blender until smooth.
6. Season with salt and black pepper to taste after adding the heavy cream and basil.

- Preparation time: 50 minutes

Dumplings and chicken

Ingredients:

- 2 tbsp unsweetened butter
- 1 chopped onion
- 2 minced garlic cloves
- 4 cup chicken stock
- 2 cups cooked chicken, chopped
- 2 peeled and sliced carrots
- 2 celery stalks, chopped
- 1 cup regular flour
- 1 tsp. baking powder
- 1 teaspoon of salt
- a half-cup of milk

Instructions:
1. Melt the butter in a big saucepan over medium heat.
2. Cook for 5-7 minutes, or until the onion is transparent, with the chopped onion and garlic.
3. Bring the chicken broth, cooked chicken, and chopped veggies to a boil in a saucepan.
4. Reduce to a low heat and cook for 20-25 minutes, or until the veggies are soft.
5. In a medium mixing basin, combine the flour, baking powder, salt, and milk to make a thick batter.
6. Drop spoonfuls of the batter into the boiling soup, cover, and continue to cook for another 15-20 minutes, or until the dumplings are cooked through.

- Preparation time: 50 minutes

Soup with Lentils

Ingredients:
- 2 tbsp of olive oil
- 1 chopped onion
- 2 minced garlic cloves
- 2 cups washed and drained dry lentils
- 4 cups veggie broth
- 2 peeled and sliced carrots
- 2 celery stalks, chopped
- 1 teaspoon thyme dried
- Season with salt and black pepper to taste.

Instructions:
1. Warm the olive oil in a big saucepan over medium heat.
2. Cook for 5-7 minutes, or until the onion is transparent, with the chopped onion and garlic.

3. Bring the dry lentils, vegetable broth, carrots, celery, thyme, salt, and black pepper to a boil in a saucepan.
4. Reduce to a low heat and cook for 45-50 minutes, or until the lentils are cooked.
- Preparation time: 50 minutes

Chowder with Clams

Ingredients:
- 4 bacon pieces, chopped
- 1 chopped onion
- 2 minced garlic cloves
- 4 quarts clam juice
- 2 gallons thick cream
- 2 peeled and sliced potatoes
- 2 cans chopped clams (6.5 ounces each)
- 1 teaspoon thyme dried
- Season with salt and black pepper to taste.

Instructions:
1. Cook the chopped bacon in a large saucepan over medium heat until crisp. Set aside the bacon using a slotted spoon.
2. Cook for 5-7 minutes, or until the onion is translucent, in the saucepan with the chopped onion and garlic.
3. Bring the clam juice, heavy cream, chopped potatoes, chopped clams, thyme, salt, and black pepper to a boil in a large saucepan.
4. Reduce to a low heat and cook for 20-25 minutes, or until the potatoes are cooked.
5. Season with salt and black pepper to taste after adding the cooked bacon.
- Preparation time: 50 minutes

Soup Minestrone

Ingredients:
- 2 tbsp of olive oil
- 1 chopped onion
- 2 minced garlic cloves
- 2 peeled and sliced carrots
- 2 celery stalks, chopped
- 1 (14.5 oz.) can chopped tomatoes, undrained
- 4 cups veggie broth
- 1 can (15 ounces) washed and drained kidney beans
- 1 sliced zucchini
- 1 tsp. dried basil
- Season with salt and black pepper to taste.

Instructions:
1. Warm the olive oil in a big saucepan over medium heat.
2. Cook for 5-7 minutes, or until the onion is transparent, with the chopped onion and garlic.
3. Bring the carrots, celery, diced tomatoes (with juice), vegetable broth, kidney beans, sliced zucchini, basil, salt, and black pepper to a boil in a large saucepan.
4. Reduce to a low heat and continue to cook for 30-35 minutes, or until the veggies are soft.
- Preparation time: 50 minutes

Soup with Chicken Tortillas

Ingredients:
- 2 tbsp of olive oil
- 1 chopped onion
- 2 minced garlic cloves
- 4 cup chicken stock
- 1 (14.5 oz.) can chopped tomatoes, undrained

- 1 can (4 ounces) drained diced green chiles
- 2 cups cooked shredded chicken
- 1 frozen cup corn
- 1 teaspoon cumin powder
- Season with salt and black pepper to taste.
- To serve, tortilla chips and shredded cheese

Instructions:
1. Warm the olive oil in a big saucepan over medium heat.
2. Cook for 5-7 minutes, or until the onion is transparent, with the chopped onion and garlic.
3. Bring to a boil the chicken broth, diced tomatoes (with juice), diced green chilies, shredded cooked chicken, frozen corn, ground cumin, salt, and black pepper.
4. Reduce the heat to low and continue to cook for 20-25 minutes, or until the flavors have merged.
5. Serve with tortilla chips and grated cheese on the side.
- Preparation time: 50 minutes

Stew with Beef

Ingredients:
- 2 pound chuck roast, sliced into 1-inch chunks
- 2 tbsp of olive oil
- 1 chopped onion
- 2 minced garlic cloves
- 4 cups beef stock
- 2 peeled and sliced carrots
- 2 celery stalks, chopped
- 2 peeled and sliced potatoes
- 1 teaspoon thyme dried
- Season with salt and black pepper to taste.

Instructions:

1.   Warm the olive oil in a big saucepan over medium
     heat.
2.   Cook for 5-7 minutes, or until the onion is transparent,
     with the chopped onion and garlic.
3.   Brown the meat cubes on both sides, approximately
     10-15 minutes.
4.   Bring the beef broth, diced carrots, celery, potatoes,
     dried thyme, salt, and black pepper to a boil in a large
     saucepan.
5.   Reduce the heat to low and continue to cook for 2-2.5
     hours, or until the meat is tender.
6.   Serve immediately.
- Preparation time: 50 minutes

Curry with Vegetables

Ingredients:
- 2 tbsp of olive oil
- 1 chopped onion
- 2 minced garlic cloves
- 1 tablespoon fresh ginger, grated
- two tbsp curry powder
- 1 (14.5 oz.) can chopped tomatoes, undrained
- 1 can (15 ounces) washed and drained chickpeas
- 2 cups chopped veggies (e.g., bell peppers, zucchini,
  eggplant)
- 1 (13.5 oz.) can coconut milk
- Season with salt and black pepper to taste.
- Serve with cooked rice

Instructions:
1.   Warm the olive oil in a big saucepan over medium
     heat.

2. Cook for 5-7 minutes, or until the onion is transparent, with the chopped onion, garlic, and grated ginger.
3. Cook for 1-2 minutes, or until the curry powder is aromatic.
4. Bring the diced tomatoes (with juice), chickpeas, chopped veggies, coconut milk, salt, and black pepper to a boil in a saucepan.
5. Reduce to a low heat and cook for 25-30 minutes, or until the veggies are soft.
6. Serve immediately over cooked rice.
- Preparation time: 50 minutes

Soup with Split Peas

Ingredients:
- 2 tbsp of olive oil
- 1 chopped onion
- 2 minced garlic cloves
- 2 cups washed and drained dry split peas
- 4 cups veggie broth
- 1 peeled and sliced carrot
- 1 celery stalk, chopped
- 1 teaspoon thyme dried
- Season with salt and black pepper to taste.

Instructions:
1. Warm the olive oil in a big saucepan over medium heat.
2. Cook for 5-7 minutes, or until the onion is transparent, with the chopped onion and garlic.
3. Bring the dried split peas, vegetable broth, carrot, celery, dried thyme, salt, and black pepper to a boil in a saucepan.

4. Reduce to a low heat and cook for 45-50 minutes, or until the split peas are cooked.
- Preparation time 50 minutes

Lentil Soup

Ingredients:
- 2 tbsp of olive oil
- 1 chopped onion
- 2 minced garlic cloves
- 2 cups washed and drained dry lentils
- 4 cups veggie broth
- 1 peeled and sliced sweet potato
- 1 chopped red bell pepper
- 1 teaspoon cumin powder
- Season with salt and black pepper to taste.

Instructions:
1. Warm the olive oil in a big saucepan over medium heat.
2. Cook for 5-7 minutes, or until the onion is transparent, with the chopped onion and garlic.
3. Bring to a boil the dry lentils, vegetable broth, chopped sweet potato, chopped red bell pepper, ground cumin, salt, and black pepper.
4. Reduce to a low heat and cook for 30-35 minutes, or until the lentils and sweet potato are cooked.
- Preparation time: 50 minutes

Soup with Tomatoes and Basil

Ingredients:
- 2 tbsp of olive oil
- 1 chopped onion

- 2 minced garlic cloves
- 2 cans chopped tomatoes, undrained (28 oz. each)
- 4 cups veggie broth
- 1/4 cup fresh basil, chopped
- Season with salt and black pepper to taste.
- Optional: grated Parmesan cheese for serving

Instructions:

1. Warm the olive oil in a big saucepan over medium heat.
2. Cook for 5-7 minutes, or until the onion is transparent, with the chopped onion and garlic.
3. Bring the diced tomatoes (with juice), vegetable broth, chopped basil, salt, and black pepper to a boil in a saucepan.
4. Reduce the heat to low and continue to cook for 20-25 minutes, or until the flavors have merged.
5. Puree the soup with an immersion blender until smooth.
6. If preferred, top with grated Parmesan cheese.

- Preparation time: 50 minutes

Dumplings and chicken

Ingredients:
- 2 tbsp of olive oil
- 1 chopped onion
- 2 minced garlic cloves
- 4 cup chicken stock
- 2 cups shredded cooked chicken
- 2 peeled and sliced carrots
- 2 celery stalks, chopped
- 1 teaspoon thyme dried
- Season with salt and black pepper to taste.

- 1 cup regular flour
- 2 tbsp. baking powder
- 1 teaspoon of salt
- 1/4 cup melted unsalted butter
- a half-cup of milk

Instructions:
1. Warm the olive oil in a big saucepan over medium heat.
2. Cook for 5-7 minutes, or until the onion is transparent, with the chopped onion and garlic.
3. Bring the chicken broth, shredded chicken, carrots, celery, dried thyme, salt, and black pepper to a boil in a large saucepan.
4. Reduce to a low heat and continue to cook for 15-20 minutes, or until the veggies are soft.
5. In a medium mixing bowl, combine the all-purpose flour, baking powder, and salt.
6. Stir in the melted butter and milk until a thick dough forms in the bowl.
7. Drop spoonfuls of the dough into the boiling soup, spacing them evenly.
8. Cook for 10-15 minutes, or until the dumplings are cooked through.

- Preparation time: 50 minutes

Soup with Beef Stroganoff

Ingredients:
- 2 tbsp. melted butter
- 1 chopped onion
- 2 minced garlic cloves
- 1 pound beef ground
- 4 cups beef stock
- 1 can condensed cream of mushroom soup (10.75 oz.)

- 1 cup mushrooms, sliced
- 1 tsp. Worcestershire sauce
- 1 teaspoon thyme dried
- Season with salt and black pepper to taste.
- 1 quart sour cream
- Freshly chopped parsley for garnish

Instructions:

1. Melt the butter in a big saucepan over medium heat.
2. Cook for 5-7 minutes, or until the onion is transparent, with the chopped onion and garlic.
3. Cook until the ground beef is browned, breaking it up with a spoon as it cooks.
4. Bring to a boil the beef broth, condensed cream of mushroom soup, sliced mushrooms, Worcestershire sauce, dried thyme, salt, and black pepper in a saucepan.
5. Reduce the heat to low and continue to cook for 20-25 minutes, or until the flavors have merged and the mushrooms are soft.
6. Remove from the heat and mix in the sour cream until completely combined.
7. Serve immediately with fresh parsley on top.
- Preparation time: 50 minutes

Stew with Black Beans and Vegetables

Ingredients:

- 2 tbsp of olive oil
- 1 chopped onion
- 2 minced garlic cloves
- 2 cans (15 oz. each) drained and washed black beans
- 2 cups veggie broth
- 1 peeled and sliced sweet potato
- 1 sliced zucchini

- 1 chopped red bell pepper
- 1 teaspoon cumin powder
- Season with salt and black pepper to taste.
- Fresh cilantro, chopped, for serving

Instructions:
1. Warm the olive oil in a big saucepan over medium heat.
2. Cook for 5-7 minutes, or until the onion is transparent, with the chopped onion and garlic.
3. Bring to a boil the black beans, vegetable broth, diced sweet potato, chopped zucchini, chopped red bell pepper, ground cumin, salt, and black pepper.
4. Reduce to a low heat and continue to cook for 30-35 minutes, or until the veggies are soft.
5. Serve immediately with fresh cilantro on top.
- Preparation time: 50 minutes

Soup with Creamy Mushrooms

Ingredients:
- 2 tbsp. melted butter
- 1 chopped onion
- 2 minced garlic cloves
- 2 cups mushrooms, sliced
- 4 cups veggie broth
- 1 quart thick cream
- 2 tbsp. all-purpose flour
- Season with salt and black pepper to taste.
- Freshly chopped parsley for garnish

Instructions:
1. Melt the butter in a big saucepan over medium heat.
2. Cook for 5-7 minutes, or until the onion is transparent, with the chopped onion and garlic.

3. Cook for 10-12 minutes, or until the sliced mushrooms have shed their moisture and are soft.
4. Bring the vegetable broth to a boil in the kettle.
5. In a small mixing bowl, combine the heavy cream and all-purpose flour.
6. Stir in the cream mixture until it is completely mixed.
7. Reduce the heat to low and continue to cook for 10-15 minutes, or until the soup has thickened and the flavors have combined.
8. Season to taste with salt and black pepper.
9. Serve immediately with fresh parsley on top.
- Preparation time: 50 minutes

Soup for an Italian Wedding

Ingredients:
- 1 pound beef ground
- 1 pound breadcrumbs
- 1/2 cup Parmesan cheese, grated
- 1 beaten egg
- 1 chopped onion
- 2 minced garlic cloves
- 8 cup chicken stock
- 1 cup tiny pasta (orzo or ditalini preferred)
- 4 cups kale, chopped
- Season with salt and black pepper to taste.
- Freshly chopped parsley for garnish

Instructions:
1. Combine the ground beef, breadcrumbs, grated Parmesan cheese, beaten egg, diced onion, and minced garlic in a large mixing bowl. To mix, integrate everything thoroughly.
2. Form the mixture into 1 inch diameter tiny meatballs.
3. Bring the chicken stock to a boil in a large saucepan.

4. Cook the meatballs in the saucepan for 10-12 minutes, or until thoroughly done.
5. Place the tiny pasta in the saucepan and simmer for 8-10 minutes, or until all dent.
6. Cook the chopped kale in the saucepan for 2-3 minutes, or until wilted.
7. Season to taste with salt and black pepper.
8. Serve immediately with fresh parsley on top.
- Preparation time: 50 minutes

Soup with Potatoes and Leek

Ingredients:
- 4 tbsp. melted butter
- 4 chopped leeks, white and light green portions only
- 3 minced garlic cloves
- 4 cup chicken stock
- 2 pounds peeled and sliced Yukon Gold potatoes
- 1 quart thick cream
- Season with salt and black pepper to taste.
- Fresh chives, chopped, for serving

Instructions:
1. Melt the butter in a big saucepan over medium heat.
2. Cook the chopped leeks and garlic for 5-7 minutes, or until the leeks are tender.
3. Bring the chicken stock and chopped potatoes to a boil in the saucepan.
4. Reduce to a low heat and cook for 25-30 minutes, or until the potatoes are soft.
5. Puree the soup with an immersion blender or in batches with a normal blender until smooth.
6. Stir in the heavy cream after returning the pureed soup to the stove.
7. Season to taste with salt and black pepper.

8. Serve immediately with fresh chives on top.
- Preparation time: 50 minutes

Soup Minestrone

Ingredients:
- 2 tbsp of olive oil
- 1 chopped onion
- 2 minced garlic cloves
- 2 celery stalks, chopped
- 2 sliced carrots
- 4 cups veggie broth
- 1 can chopped tomatoes, undrained (28 oz.)
- 1 can (15 ounces) washed and drained kidney beans
- 1 cup tiny pasta (eggplant or ditalini)
- 2 cups spinach, chopped
- 1 tsp. dried basil
- Season with salt and black pepper to taste.
- Parmesan cheese, grated, for serving

Instructions:
1. Warm the olive oil in a big saucepan over medium heat.
2. Cook for 5-7 minutes, or until the onion is transparent, with the chopped onion and garlic.
3. Cook the chopped celery and carrots for 8-10 minutes, or until the veggies are soft.
4. Bring to a boil the vegetable broth, chopped tomatoes, kidney beans, small pasta, dried basil, salt, and black pepper.
5. Reduce the heat to low and continue to cook for 20-25 minutes, or until the flavors have mingled and the pasta is soft.
6. Add the spinach to the saucepan and simmer for 2-3 minutes, or until wilted.

7. Season to taste with salt and black pepper.
8. Serve hot, topped with grated Parmesan cheese.
- Preparation time: 50 minutes

Lentil Soup

Ingredients:
- 2 tbsp of olive oil
- 1 chopped onion
- 2 minced garlic cloves
- 2 sliced carrots
- 2 celery stalks, chopped
- 2 cups lentils, dry
- 4 cups veggie broth
- 1 (14.5 oz.) can chopped tomatoes, undrained
- 1 teaspoon thyme dried
- Season with salt and black pepper to taste.
- Freshly chopped parsley for garnish

Instructions:
1. Warm the olive oil in a big saucepan over medium heat.
2. Cook for 5-7 minutes, or until the onion is transparent, with the chopped onion and garlic.
3. Cook the carrots and celery for 8-10 minutes, or until the veggies are soft.
4. Bring the dry lentils, vegetable broth, chopped tomatoes, dried thyme, salt, and black pepper to a boil in a large saucepan.
5. Reduce the heat to low and continue to cook for 30-35 minutes, or until the lentils are soft and the flavors have combined.
6. Season to taste with salt and black pepper.
7. Serve immediately with fresh parsley on top.
- Preparation time: 50 minutes

Stew with Beef

Ingredients:
- 2 tbsp of olive oil
- 2 pounds chuck meat, sliced into 1-inch chunks
- Season with salt and black pepper to taste.
- 1 chopped onion
- 3 minced garlic cloves
- 2 sliced carrots
- 2 celery stalks, chopped
- 4 cups beef stock
- 2 cups diced potatoes
- 1 cup sliced mushrooms
- 1 teaspoon thyme dried
- Freshly chopped parsley for garnish

Instructions:
1. Warm the olive oil in a large saucepan over medium-high heat.
2. Add the beef chuck to the stew and season with salt and black pepper. Cook for 5-7 minutes, or until both sides are browned.
3. Take the beef out of the saucepan and put it aside.
4. Cook for 5-7 minutes, or until the onion is translucent, in the saucepan with the chopped onion and minced garlic.
5. Cook the carrots and celery in the saucepan for 8-10 minutes, or until the veggies are soft.
6. Add the beef broth, chopped potatoes, chopped mushrooms, dried thyme, salt, and black pepper to the saucepan with the meat.

7. Bring the stew to a boil, then lower to a low heat and continue to cook for 1 1/2 to 2 hours, or until the meat is cooked.
8. Season to taste with salt and black pepper.
9. Serve immediately with fresh parsley on top.
- Preparation time: 50 minutes

Soup with Split Peas

Ingredients:
- 2 tbsp of olive oil
- 1 chopped onion
- 2 minced garlic cloves
- 2 sliced carrots
- 2 celery stalks, chopped
- 2 cups divided dried peas
- 4 cups veggie broth
- 2 c. water
- one bay leaf
- Season with salt and black pepper to taste.
- Crispy bacon to serve

Instructions:
1. Warm the olive oil in a big saucepan over medium heat.
2. Cook for 5-7 minutes, or until the onion is transparent, with the chopped onion and garlic.
3. Cook the carrots and celery for 8-10 minutes, or until the veggies are soft.
4. Bring the dried split peas, vegetable broth, water, bay leaf, salt, and black pepper to a boil in half of the kettle.
5. Reduce the heat to low and simmer for 45-50 minutes until the split peas are cooked and the soup has thickened.

6. Take the bay leaf out of the saucepan.
7. Puree the soup with an immersion blender until it reaches the desired consistency.
8. Season to taste with salt and black pepper.
9. Serve immediately with crispy bacon on top.
- Preparation time: 50 minutes

Soup with Tomatoes and Rice

Ingredients:
- 2 tbsp of olive oil
- 1 chopped onion
- 2 minced garlic cloves
- 2 sliced carrots
- 2 celery stalks, chopped
- 1 crushed tomato can (28 oz.)
- 4 cups veggie broth
- 1 cup rice, uncooked
- 1 tsp. dried basil
- Season with salt and black pepper to taste.
- Parmesan cheese, grated, for serving

Instructions:
1. Warm the olive oil in a big saucepan over medium heat.
2. Cook for 5-7 minutes, or until the onion is transparent, with the chopped onion and garlic.
3. Cook the carrots and celery for 8-10 minutes, or until the veggies are soft.
4. Bring the smashed tomatoes, vegetable broth, uncooked rice, dried basil, salt, and black pepper to a boil in a large saucepan.
5. Reduce to a low heat and continue to cook for 20-25 minutes, or until the rice is cooked and the broth has thickened.

6. Season to taste with salt and black pepper.
7. Serve hot, topped with grated Parmesan cheese.
●   Preparation time: 50 minutes.

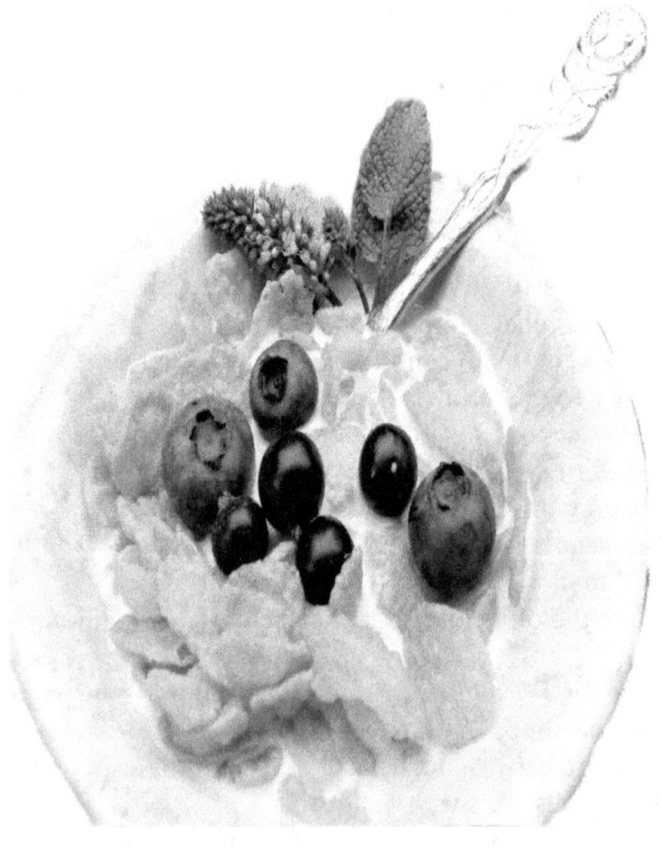

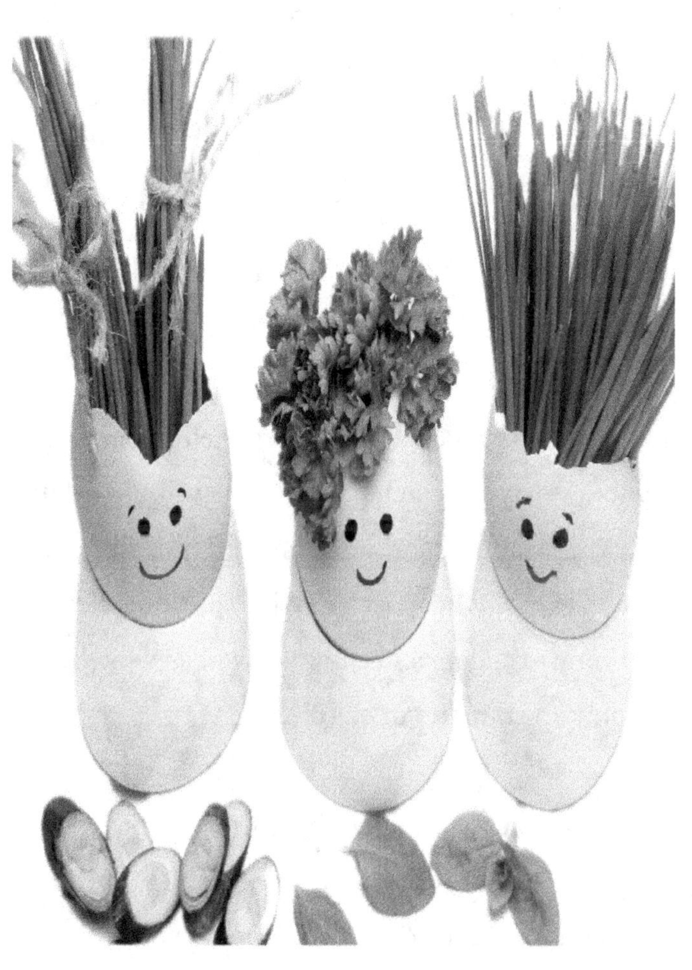

CHAPTER 7:

DIABETES DIET AVOIDABLE FOODS

Sugars and carbs that have been refined

Processed sugars and carbs have become staples in contemporary Western diets, with many individuals ingesting much too much. Although refined sugars and carbohydrates may taste delicious, they have been related to a variety of health issues, including obesity, diabetes, and heart disease. In this post, we will look at the health effects of refined sugars and carbs, as well as why they have become so common in our diets.

To begin, it is necessary to define refined sugars and carbs. Sugars that have been refined are those that have been taken from their natural source, such as cane or beet sugar, then treated to eliminate impurities. As a consequence, the product is almost all sucrose, or table sugar. Refined carbohydrates are grains that have had the bran and germ removed, leaving just the starchy endosperm. White flour and white rice are examples of such items.

Although processed sugars and carbs may taste delicious, they are really harmful to our health. When we ingest these goods, our systems swiftly break them down into glucose, which enters the circulation and causes blood sugar levels to rise rapidly. This rise in blood sugar causes the production of insulin, a hormone that aids in the absorption of glucose from the blood.

But, if we eat too much refined sugar and carbohydrates, our systems might become insulin resistant, resulting in a condition known as insulin resistance. This may eventually progress to type 2 diabetes since the body is no longer able to adequately manage its blood sugar levels.

Apart from diabetes, eating too much refined sugar and carbohydrates has been related to obesity, heart disease, and a variety of other health issues. These goods are often heavy in calories while being deficient in nutrients, resulting in overconsumption and weight gain. They also contribute to inflammation, which is a major cause of many chronic disorders.

Therefore, why have processed sugars and carbohydrates become so common in our diets? The growth of processed foods is one key issue. Many of the meals we eat today are highly processed, with added sugars and refined carbohydrates. Everything from morning cereals to granola bars to spaghetti sauce and salad dressings is included.

Another aspect is the items' broad availability. Since refined sugars and carbohydrates are inexpensive and simple to make, they are widely accessible in most grocery shops. Moreover, they are often utilized as inexpensive fillers in many packaged goods, making them even more common.

Eventually, our taste preferences come into play. Since sweet and starchy foods were formerly uncommon pleasures in our ancestors' diets, we are hardwired to seek them. In today's society, however, we have the ability to eat these foods in endless amounts, resulting in overconsumption and health issues.

Despite the hazards of ingesting too much refined sugar and carbohydrates, many individuals continue to consume these items on a daily basis. This is largely due to the addictive quality of sugar, which may make it tough to cut down or remove totally. Moreover, since sugar is typically concealed in processed meals, many individuals are unaware of how much they are ingesting.

There are many ways you may utilize to limit your consumption of processed sugars and carbohydrates. To begin, study labels and seek for hidden sugar sources such as high fructose corn syrup, dextrose, and maltodextrin. Second, prioritize whole, unprocessed foods like fruits, vegetables, and whole grains. These meals are low in sugar and abundant in nutrients, making them an excellent option for overall health.

The Consequences of Refined Carbs and Sugars

Our systems rapidly absorb refined sugars and carbohydrates, which causes a sharp increase in blood sugar levels when we ingest them. A hormone called insulin, which aids in the absorption of sugar and the utilisation of it by our cells as fuel, is released in response to this rise. Repeated blood sugar rises over time may cause insulin resistance, a disease in which our cells lose their receptivity to insulin. Type 2 diabetes may ultimately result from this disease.

Refined sugars and carbohydrates may raise the chance of developing diabetes and can cause inflammation in the body. Inflammation is a normal reaction to injury or illness, but persistent inflammation may cause a variety of health issues, including as cancer, heart disease, and stroke.

Avoid Refined Sugars and Carbs

It's important to be informed about the following when it comes to refined sugars and carbohydrates:

White sugar: This highly refined sugar is often used in soft drinks, candies, and baked products. It has minimal nutritional value and might cause inflammation and weight gain.

High-fructose corn syrup is a corn-based sweetener that is often found in processed foods like soda, candy, and baked goods. It has been associated with type 2 diabetes, insulin resistance, and a higher risk of obesity.

In baked items like bread, muffins, and pastries, white flour—a refined carbohydrate—is often used. It has minimal nutritional value and might cause inflammation and weight gain.

White rice is a refined starch that is often used in Asian cuisine. It contains little nutritional value and a lot of calories.

Soft drinks: Due to their high sugar content, these beverages may lead to weight gain, inflammation, and a higher risk of developing diabetes.

Suitable Alternatives

Thankfully, a well-balanced diet may include a variety of nutritious substitutes for processed sugars and carbohydrates. They consist of:

Whole grains may help control blood sugar levels since they are rich in fiber, vitamins, and minerals. Brown rice, quinoa, and whole wheat bread are a few examples.

Fruits: They are a natural sugar source that may fulfill a sweet appetite without raising blood sugar levels. Apples, citrus fruits, and berries are all excellent choices.

Legumes: Rich in protein and fiber, they may help control blood sugar levels. Black beans, chickpeas, and lentils are a few examples.

Nuts and seeds: They are rich in protein and good fats, and they also have the ability to control blood sugar levels. Almonds, chia seeds, and pumpkin seeds are a few examples.

Saturated and trans fatty acids

As we become older, it's more vital to pay attention to our eating patterns and make sure we're eating the proper foods in the right proportions. One source of worry is our consumption of saturated and trans fatty acids, which may be harmful to our health. In this post, we'll look at the distinctions between these two kinds of fats, their effects on our bodies, and some ways to cut down on their intake.

What is the difference between saturated and trans fatty acids?

At room temperature, saturated fatty acids are a form of fat that is solid. These can be found in animal products like meat, dairy, and eggs, as well as plant-based sources like coconut oil and palm oil. These fats may raise cholesterol levels and increase the risk of heart disease, stroke, and other health problems.

Trans fatty acids are another form of fat that might be harmful to our health. They are formed when liquid vegetable oils are partly hydrogenated, causing them to solidify. Trans fats may be present in a variety of processed meals, including fried foods, baked products, and snack items. Trans fats, like saturated fats, may raise the risk of heart disease and other health problems.

What are the effects of saturated and trans fats on human health?

A high consumption of saturated and trans fats might be harmful to our health. Eating too much of these fats may raise cholesterol levels, increasing the risk of heart disease, stroke, and other health problems.

Saturated fats have been linked to higher LDL (bad) cholesterol levels in the blood. This may contribute to the formation of plaque in the arteries, resulting in atherosclerosis and an increased risk of heart disease and stroke. Apart from these concerns, a high consumption of saturated fats may raise the chance of developing type 2 diabetes, some forms of cancer, and other chronic health problems.

Trans fats are more dangerous than saturated fats. They boost LDL cholesterol levels while decreasing HDL (good) cholesterol levels. Trans fats are also linked to inflammation in the body, which may lead to a variety of health problems such as heart disease, diabetes, and some forms of cancer.

Methods for reducing saturated and trans fat consumption

Although totally eliminating saturated and trans fats from our diets may be challenging, there are several measures we can employ to lower our consumption and lessen the detrimental effect on our health.

Choose lean proteins: When it comes to protein sources, choose lean alternatives like chicken, turkey, fish, and plant-based sources like lentils and nuts. These protein sources have less saturated and trans fats than red meat and other high-fat animal items.

Include good fats: Instead of depending on saturated and trans fats, consider including healthy fats like avocados, almonds, seeds, and olive oil into your diet. These fats may help lower cholesterol and lower the risk of heart disease.

Select low-fat dairy: When it comes to dairy products, choose for low-fat alternatives like skim milk, low-fat cheese, and nonfat yogurt. These alternatives have less saturated fat than full-fat competitors.

Minimize processed foods: Trans fats are often found in processed foods such as fried meals, baked products, and

snack foods. Reducing your consumption of these items
may help you minimize your total consumption of trans
fats.

When purchasing packaged goods, be sure to check the
nutrition label and ingredient list. Choose foods that are
low in saturated and trans fats and avoid those that include
partly hydrogenated oils or other trans fat sources.
Processed meals and foods rich in sodium

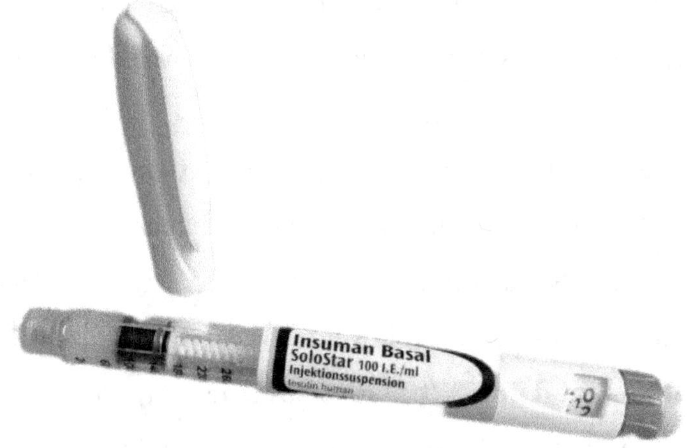

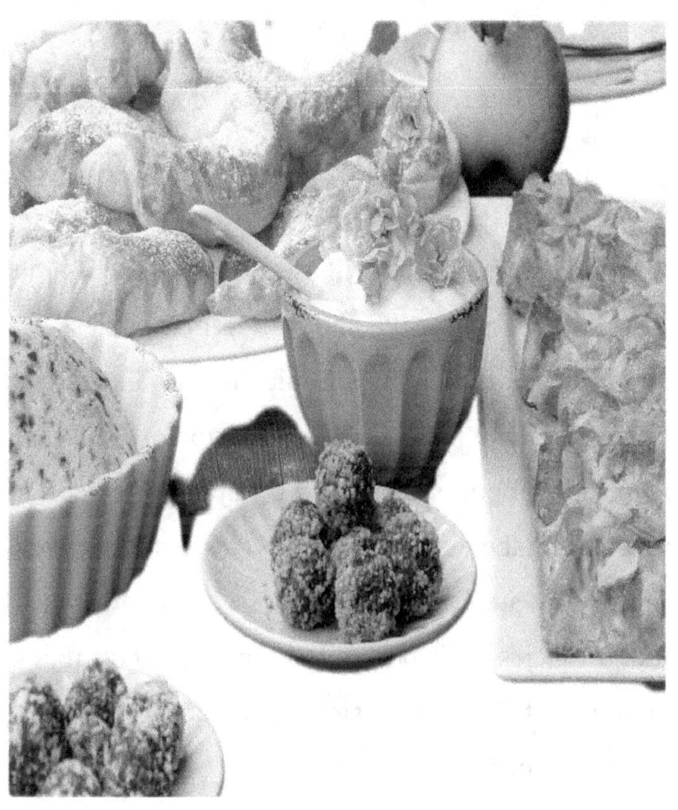

CHAPTER 8:

DIABETES TREATMENT SUGGESTIONS

Creating a support system

People typically need additional assistance as they age in order to preserve their health and well-being. This is especially true for those with chronic diseases like diabetes, who may struggle to manage their condition on their own. Establishing a support system may be an important component of diabetes care beyond 50, assisting people in remaining motivated, tracking progress, and addressing potential obstacles. This post will go through ways for developing a solid support system for diabetes control beyond the age of 50.

- **Friends and family**

  Family and friends are one of the most significant sources of support for people with diabetes. Family and friends may provide emotional support, encouragement, and help with duties such as food

shopping and meal preparation. They may also help
people remain on track with their diabetes control
objectives by checking in on a frequent basis and
providing inspiration.

- **Diabetes Support Organizations**
Joining a diabetic support group might help people
connect with others who are going through similar
circumstances. These groups might be found in
local hospitals, community centers, or online
forums. They provide a chance to exchange
diabetes-management experiences, advice, and
techniques, as well as emotional support and a
feeling of community.

- **Educators in Diabetes**
Diabetes educators are educated individuals who
can give diabetes education and assistance.
Individual or group sessions may be provided to
assist people with diabetes understand their disease,
build a tailored care plan, and learn practices for

balanced food, physical exercise, and medication control. Diabetes instructors may be found at healthcare facilities, hospitals, or community centers.

- **Healthcare Professionals**

Frequent visits to healthcare professionals may be an important part of diabetes control beyond the age of 50. These experts can advise you on diabetes care options, prescription modifications, and blood sugar monitoring. They may also answer any concerns or queries people have regarding their condition.

- **Dietitians and nutritionists**

Healthy eating is an important part of diabetes care, and engaging with a nutritionist or dietitian may assist in designing a meal plan that is tailored to an individual's specific requirements. These specialists may advise on portion sizes, food selections, and dietary techniques for controlling blood sugar levels.

- **Partners for Exercise**

  Physical activity is an important element of diabetes control, and having a workout partner may help people remain motivated and responsible. A workout partner may give motivation, assist in setting and achieving objectives, and make exercise more pleasurable.

- **Technology**

  Those with diabetes now have a new method to get help because to advances in technology. Individuals may use mobile applications and internet platforms to measure their blood sugar levels, manage their food consumption, and get prescription reminders. These tools may be especially beneficial for those who do not have access to in-person assistance or prefer to manage their diabetes on their own.

The significance of frequent check-ups and screenings

People's bodies alter as they age, increasing the probability of experiencing health problems. This is why, beyond the age of 50, regular check-ups and screenings become even more important. In this post, we will explore the need of regular check-ups and screenings, which tests to prioritize, and how often visits should be scheduled.

Why are frequent check-ups and screenings necessary beyond the age of 50?

Diabetes, high blood pressure, heart disease, and certain kinds of cancer may not display symptoms in the early stages. Frequent check-ups and screenings may aid in the early detection of many disorders, when they are more curable and controllable.

Chronic illnesses such as diabetes, heart disease, and cancer are among the primary causes of mortality among older persons. You can avoid and treat these diseases by routinely checking your health.

Keeping track of prescriptions and treatments: To manage chronic diseases, older persons are often given many medications. Frequent visits to your doctor may help you remain on top of your prescriptions and verify they are functioning properly.

Check-ins for mental health: Older persons are also at risk of acquiring mental health problems such as depression and anxiety. Frequent check-ins with a mental health expert may assist in identifying and treating these problems before they worsen.

Which tests should be given top priority?

High blood pressure, often known as hypertension, is a frequent problem in older persons and may raise the risk of heart disease and stroke. Blood pressure checks should be performed at least once a year.

Cholesterol: Elevated cholesterol levels may raise the risk of heart disease. Men over 45 and women over 55 should get their cholesterol levels examined every five years at the absolute least.

Diabetes: Elderly persons are more likely to acquire type 2 diabetes. Blood sugar levels should be examined at least once every three years, and more often if diabetes runs in the family.

Colorectal cancer is the third most prevalent malignancy in older persons. Screening for this malignancy should begin at the age of 50 and may be accomplished by a variety of procedures including colonoscopies, fecal occult blood tests, and stool DNA testing.

Breast cancer screening: Mammograms should be performed on women over the age of 50 to test for breast cancer.

Prostate cancer screening: Men over the age of 50 should get frequent prostate cancer screenings, which may involve a PSA blood test and a digital rectal exam.

How often should check-ups and screenings be performed?

Blood pressure checks should be done at least once a year, as previously stated.

Cholesterol levels should be examined at least every five years, or more regularly if they are high or there is a family history of heart disease.

Diabetes: Blood sugar levels should be examined at least once every three years, or more regularly if diabetes runs in the family or if you have additional risk factors such as obesity or high blood pressure.

Colorectal cancer screening should begin at the age of 50 and be repeated every 5-10 years, depending on the technique employed and the results of prior screens.

Breast cancer: Mammograms should be performed every two years on women over the age of 50.

Prostate cancer: Men over the age of 50 should consult with their doctor to determine the optimum screening plan for them.

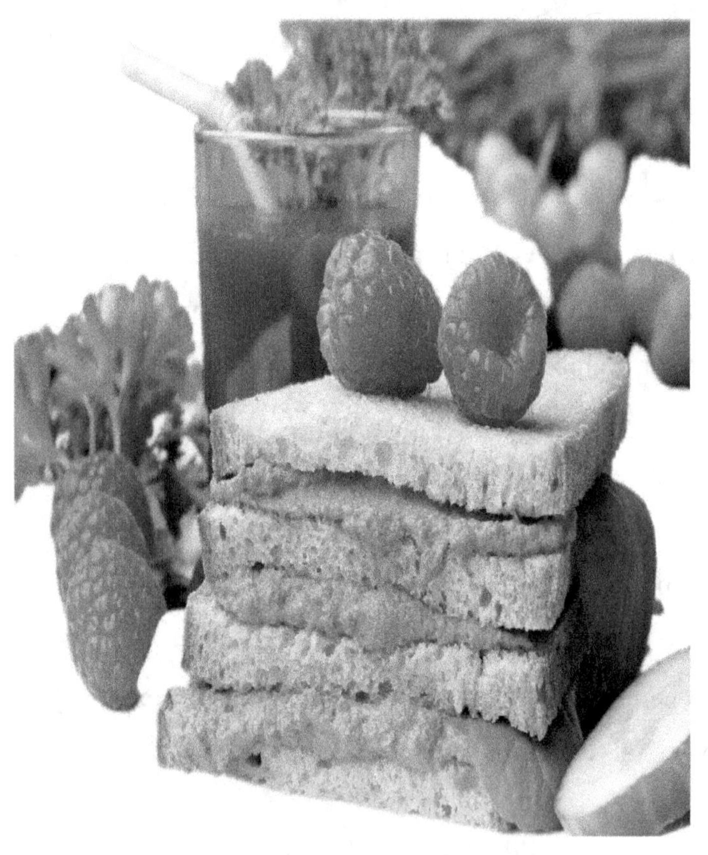

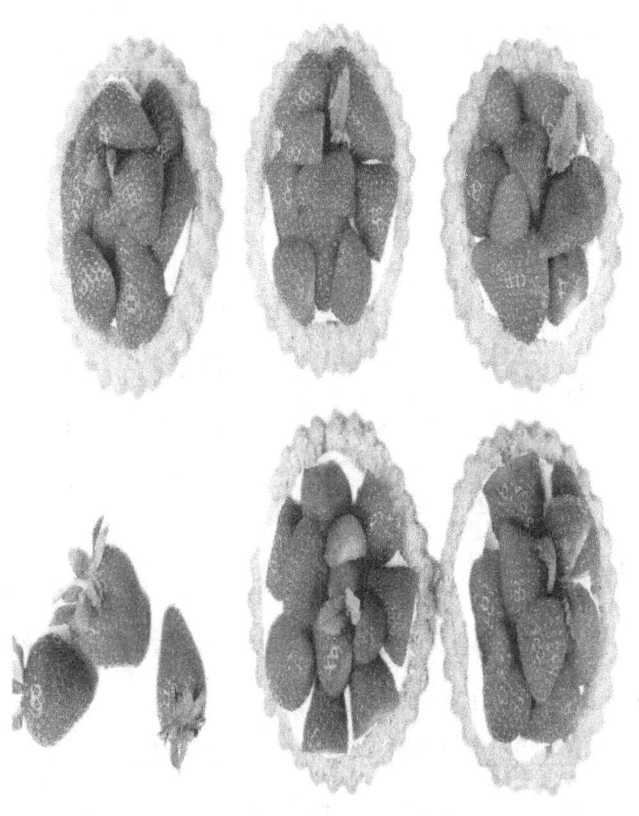

CHAPTER 9:

CONCLUSION AND FURTHER RESOURCES

A summary of the main points

Our bodies change as we age, including changes in metabolism, which may contribute to the beginning of a variety of health problems, including diabetes. Diabetes management beyond the age of 50 might be difficult, but it is vital to maintain a healthy and active lifestyle to avoid complications.

Maintaining a well-balanced diet that satisfies the body's nutritional demands while keeping blood sugar levels in line is one of the most important parts of diabetes care after 50. Complex carbs, whole grains, healthy fats, lean proteins, and fruits and vegetables should be included in the diet, but processed sugars and carbohydrates should be avoided.

Meal planning is an important element of diabetes treatment since it entails selecting the proper meals in the right amounts. Meal planning ahead of time may help you make healthier choices and prevent impulsive decisions that can lead to bad eating habits. A well-planned dinner may also help you save time and minimize stress in your day-to-day life.

Apart from meal preparation, it is important to keep hydrated throughout the day by consuming enough of water and other fluids. It is also critical to avoid alcohol and restrict caffeine use, since both may alter blood sugar levels.

Frequent physical exercise is essential for overall health and blood sugar regulation. Physical exercise may increase insulin sensitivity, blood sugar levels, and general health. It is advised to participate in moderate activity for at least 30 minutes each day, five days per week. Brisk walking, swimming, cycling, and strength training are all healthy activities.

Stress management is also an important element of diabetes care beyond the age of 50. Persistent stress may cause the production of hormones that impact blood sugar levels, thus stress should be managed using a variety of approaches such as deep breathing, meditation, yoga, and frequent exercise.

It is critical to monitor blood sugar levels on a regular basis and to have frequent check-ups and screenings to identify and treat any possible issues. Blood pressure, cholesterol levels, and renal function may all be monitored. To build a tailored diabetes treatment plan, it is also critical to collaborate closely with a healthcare team that includes a primary care physician, endocrinologist, and registered dietitian.

Establishing a support system may also help with diabetes management beyond the age of 50. This includes family, friends, and support groups. It is critical to talk freely and honestly with loved ones about the problems of diabetes management and to solicit their assistance when necessary.

Further diabetes management and support resources

Diabetes management may be difficult, particularly for elderly people. Luckily, numerous services are available to assist seniors in managing their diabetes and living a healthy, meaningful life. Educational publications, support groups, food planning tools, and physical activity programs are all examples of resources. This post will go over some of the top diabetes management and support options for seniors over the age of 50.

Diabetes Association of America (ADA)

The American Diabetes Association (ADA) is a non-profit organization that promotes diabetes education, support, and advocacy. Their website is a comprehensive source of diabetes management information, including information on healthy food, physical exercise, medication management, and other topics. In addition, they provide a number of online tools and resources, such as meal planning guidelines, blood glucose monitors, and self-assessment quizzes. Moreover, the ADA offers chances for seniors to engage with other diabetics via support groups and community activities.

Medicare

Medicare is a government health insurance program for those 65 and older, as well as some disabled younger people. Diabetes-related services covered by Medicare include diabetes screening tests, diabetes education, and medical supplies. It is critical for diabetic elders to understand what Medicare covers and how to get these treatments.

Diabetes and Digestive and Kidney Disorders National Institute (NIDDK)

The NIDDK is a branch of the National Institutes of Health (NIH) that undertakes diabetes and other health-related research. This website has a variety of diabetes care information, including tips on good diet, physical exercise, and medication administration. They also give information on the most recent diabetes research as well as diabetic management advice.

The DPP is a lifestyle modification program designed to prevent or postpone the development of type 2 diabetes. The program is intended for adults who are at risk of getting diabetes and focuses on good food, physical exercise, and weight reduction. The program has been demonstrated to reduce the risk of diabetes in persons over the age of 60 by 58%.

Diabetes Self-Management Help and Education (DSMES) DSMES is a program that offers diabetes education and assistance to individuals. Healthy nutrition, physical exercise, medication management, and blood glucose monitoring are among the topics covered in the curriculum. DSMES is generally offered in a group or individual setting by trained diabetes educators. Diabetes patients are covered by Medicare for DSMES.

Resources available in the local community

Local community services may be an excellent source of assistance for diabetic elders. Support groups, fitness programs, and healthy cooking classes are examples of such resources. See what services are available in your region by contacting your local elder center, community center, or hospital.